VICTORY OVER CANCER!
VOL 2

VICTORY OVER CANCER!
VOL 2

Acid Reflux and Esophageal Cancer

By Joseph Marx

An Imprint of Joseph Marx
Mary Esther, Florida

Book Edited by Kelly Marx, B.A. Journalism, GWU

An Imprint of Joseph Marx, Mary Esther, Florida
ISBN 10-0998352268
Victoryovercancer.org

The names used in this book are spelled out only by prior permission; otherwise all other names are represented by a single capital letter.

PREFACE

Victory Over Cancer: Vol 2, like Vol 1, has one key objective, and that is to share information that is not widely known, with those who want to prevent cancer, or who have cancer and are desperate to survive it. Volume 2 extends the information of Volume 1 into a more in-depth discussion on how to cure chronic acid reflux, its progression to Barrett's Esophagus, Dysplasia, Esophageal Cancer and Laryngo-pharyngeal Cancer, and the various treatment options for all of these conditions.

Certain critical pieces of information in this book are buried in scientific studies to the extent that many in the medical profession are unaware of them, let alone the average cancer patient. Not a single one of the numerous oncology doctors and nurses I have had over the last five years knew of the metabolic weaknesses of cancer, nor did they understand that these weaknesses could be exploited smartly with diet in a safe manner that empowers a cancer patient to potentially slow their tumor's rate of growth and even reverse it. Some of the medical people I approached with my findings were very open minded and wanted to research the topic further. Others appeared to become put-off that a layperson could possibly know something about cancer that the average doctor doesn't know—I suppose they thought I was a buffoon, peddling a quack remedy based on pseudoscience. They are wrong on every account. I'm simply some one who wants to survive their cancer, when conventional medicine doesn't have the answer. It brought me back to the first Planet of the Apes movie, when Charlton Heston speaks to the Apes for the first time. The Apes were in disbelief—humans are not supposed to be able to talk. I guess I am not supposed to be able to research scientific journals, think critically, and apply new information in a manner that might save my life.

In any case, there is much more in this book that will help someone to not only prevent cancer, but also help cancer patients get organized, navigate through the complicated cancer treatment matrix, make difficult treatment decisions, learn about numerous safe things they can do at home to improve their chance of survival, and learn about alternative and integrative cancer treatment options that can be powerful adjuncts to any type of cancer treatment program.

ACKNOWLEDGMENTS

I am deeply thankful to my wife Kelly for editing Volume 2 of this book, and who encouraged me every step of the way to share my story so that others might find hope and a safer and more natural path to recovery.

CONTENTS

INTRODUCTION

If you or a loved one has recently been diagnosed with cancer, then you are in a life-altering situation. The author found himself in such a crisis in September 2013. After years of living with chronic acid reflux, he discovered he had a very deadly cancer and set himself on a quest to be healed. This book is a story about his insufferable journey with cancer. It reveals numerous scientifically based things cancer patients can do safely at home, to improve their odds of winning their battle with cancer. These are things the author discovered along the way that he wishes he had known much earlier. He is sharing this information in the hope that it will significantly reduce the suffering of many, and prolong their lives beyond anything conventional treatment can provide alone.

What distinguishes this book is that the author exposes things that are little known by most people and are not part of the national discussion, nor are they a part of the conventional cancer treatment system. Although the author is not part of the medical profession, he has an extensive background in science and mathematics, and has spent a good part of his professional career teaching, researching, and writing about technical subjects. The discoveries in this book are carefully broken down into a context that is easy to understand.

When someone experiences a bone jarring collision with cancer, they all ask the same question. What do I do now? Such a simple question begs for a simple answer. Simple answers however, are oftentimes mockingly elusive. Instead of a simple answer, most find themselves immersed in a massive and convoluted maze of information, with no clear answers and nowhere to turn. For each question that is answered, five more pop up. For those overwhelmed by indecision and lack of knowledge, this book will empower them to boldly take control of their treatment plan. They will be shown clear steps to take immediately.

Concurrent with a crisis of information overload, every patient is confronted with the reality that every single day it takes to get into treatment, the cancer continues to grow at an alarming rate, frequently eight to 15 times faster than normal cells. In hyper metabolic cancers the growth rate is out of control. Tumors have no switches to turn off––or cords to pull—or circuits to break. Something needs to intervene on the patient's behalf to stop the tumor from invading every area of the body and starving the patient to death. Every day the patient waits to get into treatment matters—and it matters a lot. Just think of what someone's outcome might be if they were able to reduce the rate of growth of their tumor or even stop it dead in its track, prior to entering treatment. This book provides scientifically proven countermeasures that speak powerfully to this problem and also the problem of preventing recurrence. Such is the cornerstone of this book—to empower patients with knowledge that may make the difference between life and death.

The author uncovers various natural and holistic antidotes that cancer patients can do immediately to attack their cancer, slow its rate of growth, and potentially reverse its growth and even cure it, using nutritional therapy, therapeutic levels of exercise, and targeted natural substances. He carefully dissects the science underpinning an anticancer diet that exploits the metabolic abnormalities of cancer that have been neglected in the war against cancer, and on its own, has the potential to substantially improve a patient's outcome. If this diet is implemented prior to the time a patient enters treatment, it is entirely possible for the patient to downgrade their tumor. A downgraded tumor means the treatment has a much greater chance of being effective. When these natural and holistic antidotes are added to a conventional, integrative or alternative cancer treatment regimen, they produce a prescription for an optimal outcome.

The reader will also find extensive discussions on: two key contributors to cancer, poor digestion and chronic inflammation—the harshness of conventional treatment—the value of an alkaline diet—how sodium bicarbonate can be used as a weapon against cancer—how to fortify the body to prevent recurrence—what to do if it comes back–

–conventional and alternative Immunotherapy and where to find it— how alternative Immunotherapy differs from conventional Immunotherapy—and the danger of circulating cancer stem cells and what can be done about it. It also reveals novel early detection cancer blood tests that are not offered by conventional medicine, namely, chemo sensitivity testing and natural substance sensitivity testing, along with information on where to get these tests. Also included is a list of extensively researched alternative cancer treatment centers that are available in the United States. This book will save patients hundreds of hours of research trying to sort through the vast amount of information on the Internet, as well as equip them with enough knowledge to provide a departure point for exploring safer alternative or integrative options as complements to conventional treatment, especially when conventional treatment fails the patient.

In sum, the holistic prescriptions in this book not only attack cancer prior to treatment and make the treatment more effective, they reduce the side effects of chemo, radiation and surgery, help the patient prevent recurrence, and afford the patient a realistic alternative cancer treatment option if they should fail conventional treatment.

Too many people are needlessly dying of cancer, who would have lived longer if they had been equipped with the right information. In this regard, knowledge is power. This book will empower you with the freedom to take control of your cancer and live. Are you ready? Let's take a closer look and learn how to have victory over cancer!

CHAPTER 1

The Sabbatical

Come to me, all you who labor and are
heavy laden, and I will give you rest.
—Matthew 11:28

As quickly as I lost consciousness I recovered from one of those deep and pleasant sleeps. As I lay on my left side, draped in white sheets, I detected a faint sound slowly beeping in my right ear. My eyes reluctantly peeked open and formed into narrow slits—like cats do as they purr themselves into a catatonic state. Still under the spell of the Propofol, I became greedy to fall back into that luscious sleep. Rest is all I wanted on Anna Maria Island.

Suddenly, I felt someone pat both sides of my face saying, "Joe, wake up, Joe, it's time to wake up." My eyes opened wider this time and the lights in the recovery room hit me like headlights from a semi truck at night. Sitting at the bedside and slanting towards me is Doctor E., my Gastroenterologist. Doctor E. is in his mid-thirties, well groomed, with dark wavy hair tucked under a hair net, and is wearing pale green scrubs. An ivory-white mask lay unassumingly over his neck and photos of the procedure rested in his lap. Kelly is slightly to his left, peering at me with her big toothy smile as if everything is fine.

Touching my shoulder, Doctor E. asked, "How are you feeling?" I said, "Pretty good, I feel like I'm starting to wake up really fast." He said, "Yes, Propofol doesn't knock you out so hard. Most patients come out of it pretty fast." I drifted off a little and remember thinking, "Isn't this one of the drugs Michael Jackson supposedly overdosed on? Now I understand why it's used as a sleep aid." However, Propofol wasn't the sort of rest I was longing for.

Three days prior, on September 9th, 2013, was the day Kelly and I arrived at Bradenton Beach on Anna Maria Island, along the Gulf Coast of Florida. We had just completed a year in Jacksonville, Florida, after having moved from Colorado the year prior. The last of our four children had moved out and we were empty nesters. The time for relocation to warmer weather had arrived. It also placed us within an easy drive of our oldest daughter and her family.

Kelly was much more nervous about the move then I was. Nonetheless, we both yearned for a hotter climate and more time with our grandkids, and this swayed her to make the warm-weather leap. As soon as we got to Florida I plunged head first into a really bad Middle School teaching assignment. Previously, I taught mostly High School. The new job proved to be a monumental mistake. I showed up expecting to have Standard Math kids. At least this is what I was told in the interview. Instead, they gave me six low performing classes with a mix of special needs children in two of them. Public schools can be terribly abusive of teachers new to their district. As the year wore on, Kelly made a point of reminding me how exhausted I looked all the time. Kelly and all four of our kids urged me to quit midyear but I didn't listen. Instead, I decided I would be the good soldier and gut it out. At the end of the school year, I finally came to my senses. I decided to quit teaching after 11 years, as a second career. I desperately needed a sabbatical.

Staying in Jacksonville was not an option. The poor job experience put a sour taste in my mouth for that area. Kelly was also extremely frustrated trying to find something other than part time work in Jacksonville. We had previously visited Anna Maria Island on a number of occasions and fell in love with it. We both thought it would be a terrific place to take a respite from the stresses of life. It is just north of Sarasota on the Gulf Coast. The community is small with a lot of year round residents. It reminded us of the small towns we both lived in as kids. It would also keep us within a day's drive of our grandkids. Besides, the white sandy-beaches and semi-tropical climate are irresistible. We decided we could try it out and perhaps make it our permanent home.

We put everything into storage in Jacksonville, and then signed a three-month lease on a fully furnished apartment no more than 75 yards from the ocean. If we decided to stay, Kelly could work part time as a dental hygienist and I could possibly teach Math at one of the local

Colleges. So Anna Maria Island became an oasis on the horizon to us, a place where we could quench our thirst for rest, reinvigorate our marriage, and refocus our lives. We expected good fortune at an oasis but something else seemed to be happening the night we drove down.

It was Monday, September 9th, only an hour after leaving Jacksonville when I became brutally sick to my stomach. It came on so sudden that I remember pondering whether it was food poisoning. We pulled into our white and yellow trimmed apartment around 9:30 pm under a light rain and fog. The ocean was so close we could hear the waves breaking and smell the salt water, while we unpacked the cars. Soon after going to bed I found myself in the bathroom retching with the dry heaves, and subsequently blacked out as I tried to exit the bathroom. I had never passed out before and this scared the heck out of Kelly.

The next morning welcomed us with sunny skies, 80 degrees of low humidity air, and a placid ocean. I was also feeling better. We quickly immersed ourselves into the beach and the ocean and enjoyed the day despite the annoyance of what transpired the night before. By Wednesday however, I had experienced two days of pitch-black stools, usually a sign of an internal bleed. I remember sitting in the emergency room (ER) on day three of our sabbatical thinking, "What in the world is happening? I just finished the worse job of my life and now I'm in the ER three days into our sabbatical." The ER Doctor suspected I had a bleeding ulcer, especially after I told him about the stressful job and the wheel barrel of Tums I had consumed over the last 20 or so years. He admitted me to the hospital and ordered an upper endoscopy first thing the next morning. Doctor E. would be my Gastroenterologist.

Gastroenterologists specialize in the digestive tract, which includes the esophagus, stomach, colon, rectum, liver, pancreas and gallbladder. Other organs of the digestive system include the mouth, tongue, salivary glands, and pharynx (throat), but are treated by other doctors. By the way, all of these organs come with some of the most dangerous cancers, and all of them are connected to digestive disorders in some fashion. More and more science is showing that most diseases, in one way or another, can be traced back to some sort of digestive issue.

Doctor E. would perform a procedure called an upper endoscopy, which is a technique used to examine the inside of the upper digestive tract using an endoscope. The endoscope is a thin-flexible tube, with a high-resolution fiber optic camera. Tiny instruments are attached to it.

The Doctor examines everything in the throat, esophagus, stomach, and upper part of the small intestine.

The hospital Internist, Doctor T., explained the procedure in detail. She said, "We suspect it's a bleeding ulcer, but don't worry it's a very safe procedure. The doctor will find the bleed and stop it. He can also remove any suspicious tissue and biopsy it." I had never really thought about the possibility of something more than a bleeding stomach ulcer, but I sensed something else was wrong. She mentioned the term esophagus, a term I had not heard in a long time.

The esophagus is commonly known as the food pipe. It's a tube that starts where the throat ends in the lower part of the neck, at the junction of the larynx and voice box. The larynx is actually a small tube that connects the throat to the windpipe. The esophagus then passes behind the lungs and heart and through the diaphragm, a flat muscle between the lungs and stomach that is used for breathing. It is typically 8 to 10 inches long. The esophagus is used to transport food and fluids from the throat to the stomach using muscular contractions.[1] The following is an illustration of the upper digestive anatomy of a human.

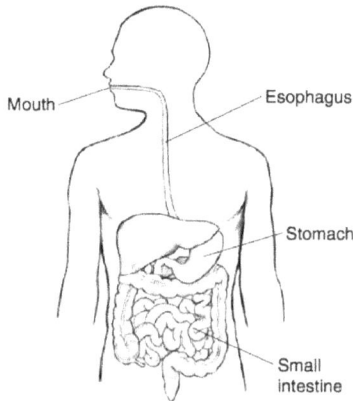

Upper Digestive Anatomy[2]

Looking Under the Hood

A nurse with a cheery smile woke me up at 5:00 am to take blood, check my vitals and prep me for the upcoming procedure at 7:30 am. From that point on time seemed to speed up. Soon I was on a hospital gurney trundling down passageways, through swinging doors, coming to rest in a pre-surgical bay. Doctor E. swung by for a short visit saying, "The procedure should take no more than 15 to 20 minutes and I'll debrief you and Kelly afterward in the recovery room." As I lay there, the last thing I remember hearing was a nurse saying, "I just administered the anesthesia into your IV and you should start feeling sleepy in 15 to 20 seconds."

No sooner had my lights turned out and I was waking up to Doctor E. and Kelly at my bedside. "You did really well with the procedure," he said, "but I was surprised to find a large mass located at the junction of the lower esophagus and the stomach with a tear in it, called a Mallory Weiss tear. I cauterized the tear but had to use a clip because of severe inflammation around the tear. The clip will dissolve on its own." After he said these words, I sensed my life was about to change as abruptly as I woke up.

Doctor E. then extended several color pictures of the procedure towards me, pointed and said, "Your esophagus is badly damaged from exposure to stomach acid and it looks like you've had this condition for years. You need to immediately start taking some medication to reduce stomach acid." He also gave me a list of lifestyle and diet changes that I needed to adapt as soon as possible to help the esophagus heal. I asked, "What are the chances that it's cancerous?" He said, "I believe it's primarily inflammation, but I took multiple biopsies and will personally visit pathology and get the results to you as soon as possible. I also want to see you first thing next week." I wondered how a mass had grown on my lower esophagus for who-knows how long, with no pain or other indications it was there? It was awfully disconcerting.

Within days following the endoscopy Doctor E. called with some good news. He said, "Pathology determined the biopsies are negative! However, you still have a mass at the lower esophagus that is highly inflamed from years of acid reflux." So he put me on a Proton Pump Inhibitor (PPI), called Protonix, which is a strong prescription drug used to reduce stomach acid by blocking the enzyme in the wall of the stomach that produces acid. Doctor E. made it clear that it would take a lot of effort on my part to make some significant changes to diet and lifestyle to bring the inflammation down."

Kelly and I both knew the stressful teaching job pushed my health over the edge, yet it seemed I was in some type of stressful job my entire adult life. I remembered all of the stressful jobs I had while I was in the military—the many sleepless nights and gallons of coffee—the constant indigestion. The Western work ethic allows us to accomplish many things in life, but it can also provide a noose to hang ourselves with if we let it. Perhaps stress not only triggered poor eating habits, but also depreciated my immune system. In fact, the hospital Internist commented, "I believe the primary cause of your digestive disorder is stress." Extremely stressful life situations, particularly unbearable job situations, or toxic relationships for long periods of time are key trigger events for all kinds of bad health. Please do not do what I did. Find a new job before it tries to kill you.

Although our fortune had not faired well in Florida, we refused to let it upend our plan to immerse ourselves in some rest. To try and bring a little perspective to our situation, I remember saying to Kelly, "What better occasion to have a medical emergency then on the day we start a sabbatical."

A Few More Surprises

During the one-week follow-up Doctor E. reviewed my medical history and treatment plan. Kelly accompanied me, as she would continue to do throughout all of my future appointments. We shook hands as we entered his tidy and well-lit office, made some small talk, and sat down. Behind him was a large computer screen with pictures he took of the procedure. He sat down in a padded black-leather office chair, placed my medical records from Colorado in his lap and began to page through them. He asked, "How long have you been in Bradenton?" I said, "Barely a week." He responded, "You're kidding? Are you on vacation here?" Then I gave him the lowdown on my most recent job experience, and why we were in Bradenton. He nodded as I spoke, then wheeled his chair closer, leaned forward, and asked some questions about my medical history. "Are you on any medications for GERD right now?" I said, "I'm not on any medications except I've been taking Tums for years. What's GERD?" With a puzzled look, he asked, "You've never been diagnosed with GERD?" "No," I said, "I've never heard of it." He explained that GERD stands for Gastrointestinal-Esophageal Reflux Disease and that it is much more than heartburn. It is synonymous with acid reflux, where reflux means pushing up into the esophagus—something I never knew. Acid reflux can cause the cells in the lining of the esophagus to transform themselves into quasi stomach cells, which can become pre-cancerous and even progress to cancer. The chances of it progressing to cancer are small, but if it does, it can be extremely dangerous because it's not normally detected until it's well advanced and blocks the passage of food. This was a lot for us to digest.

Doctor E. wanted to hear more about the Tums. I explained, "I take them frequently. I always have a small pack of Tums in my pocket, glove compartment, book bag, desk at school and nightstand." He asked, "Why haven't you discussed this with your primary care physician?" I said, "I got use to heartburn. It seemed like a normal part of life."

After I finished speaking, he pointed at a spot on a photo and explained, "You have an anatomical condition called a Sliding Hiatal Hernia." I said, "I've never heard of it." He continued, "It's a condition where part of the stomach pushes past the diaphragm into the lung cavity, and gets temporarily strangulated." I said, "I thought a hernia is a tear in the abdominal wall?" He responded, "A hiatal hernia is not a tear, but it is a causative factor in acid reflux. It inhibits the lower sphincter muscle of the esophagus from properly closing, which permits stomach acid to seep into the esophagus."

He also pointed out that everyone who has a hiatal hernia doesn't necessarily have GERD, but everyone who has GERD has a hiatal hernia. The missing shards to my broken medical history came together. Before leaving his office, he encouraged me to take responsibility for the treatment plan, which included changes to diet and eating habits. He didn't use the word cancer, but I got the general idea. After leaving his office, Kelly and I quickly decided that the worst was over—or, at least that's what we thought.

Back To The Main Thing

Anna Maria Island is a barrier island with sugary-white beaches that stretch seven miles along the west coast of Florida, just north of Sarasota and south of Saint Petersburg. We were in the Bradenton Beach area, on the southern portion of the Island. The small communities on Anna Maria Island remain relatively untouched from commercial development, something not easy to find in Florida. Along the public beach areas, traffic can get a little crowded during the peak season from November to June. Yet, there are plenty of sparsely populated spots if you don't mind walking a little from the public parking areas, which are free of charge. They even have a free public trolley that provides transportation from the north end of the Island all the way south to Longboat Key and Sarasota. There are plenty of small shops and restaurants peppered along the Island with spectacular views of the ocean. The marine wildlife and fishing is some of the best in Florida, including a large population of manatees, which look like over-stuffed seals with huge fan-like tails. They swim throughout the bays and inlets. Numerous natural preserves also surround the Island. Several times a day, dolphins swam by our beach in groups of two to four, sometimes within 10 yards of the beach, unfazed by any bathers near by, as if bidding us a fair day. During our first weeks, especially in the morning there were literally no breaking waves along the shore. Calm waters cuddled up to the shore. We found rest.

The Fish That Caught Me

One of the first things I did after leaving Doctor E.'s office was to buy some saltwater fishing rods and gear. That next morning I went fishing. I spent the first few hours without a single bite. Then something amazing happened—at least as it goes, in the mind of a fisherman. Recorded from my Journal, September 16, 2013:

I caught my first fish on Bradenton Beach but in a very peculiar way. It was a 17-inch mackerel. I reeled him in and noticed a brand new golden lure hooked on the corner of his mouth; but it wasn't the silver lure that I was using. I was puzzled until I realized that the lure in its mouth got tangled in my fishing line as he swam by. His hook caught my line, not the other way around. I used this golden lure the rest of the morning and caught numerous fish with it. It became my good luck lure. I thanked God.

I went on to fish with this same lure in the coming weeks and caught multiple fish with it, returning them all back to the ocean in honor of the friendly mackerel—and the sabbatical was splendid.

Notes

1. WebMD, Digestive Disorders Health Center, http://www.webmd.com/digestive-disorders/picture-of-the-esophagus (accessed March 4, 2015, 1).
2. National Institute of Diabetes and Digestive and Kidney Diseases, Barrett's Esophagus.pdf document Illustration, http://www.niddk.nih.gov/health-information/health-topics/digestive-diseases/barretts-esophagus/Documents/barretts_508.pdf (accessed March 4, 2015, 1).

CHAPTER 2

Acid Reflux And Cancer

It is a very bad habit to put off disagreeable things.
—Alain de Botton

Within days of my hospital visit I found myself in a delightful situation, waste deep in the Gulf of Mexico, soaking up the sun while swinging a fiberglass fishing rod over my head. I was determined to not let a little bump in the road with my health interrupt the sabbatical. As I gathered my equipment to search for a more productive fishing spot, my back started to itch as if someone added poison ivy extract to my sun tan lotion. So I decided to scoot back to the apartment. Kelly quickly determined that I had hives and was allergic to the Proton Pump Inhibitor. In a strange way the hives reeled me back into the reality that I had a more serious health issue going on then I was willing to admit. Since the biopsy was negative I felt the whole episode wasn't a big deal anymore. Nothing could be farther from the truth. I finally accepted this fact and decided it was time to get smart on digestive diseases.

One of the first things I learned is the deadly link between chronic acid reflux and esophageal cancer, and laryngopharyngeal cancer (known as voice box and throat cancer).[1] Most who have chronic acid reflux do not fully appreciate how serious the risk is that it might one day progress into a serious gastro condition followed by cancer.

At any rate, the focus of this chapter is to bring desperately needed awareness to the deadly link between chronic acid reflux and its progression to cancer, something few people are aware of. It will also bring awareness to numerous digestive related diseases that lead to cancer, which are among the most deadly types of cancer.

With millions of people in the United States experiencing acid reflux at least one to two times a week; it's time to get the word out. Even if you do not have acid reflux or a gastrointestinal related disease, I hope you find this chapter helpful in learning the truth about acid reflux's deadly link to cancer. Let's first take a look at digestive diseases and cancer.

DIGESTIVE DISEASE AND CANCER

Numerous naturopathic and holistic health experts believe that a damaged digestive system is the source of many, if not most diseases and disorders of the body. This view contradicts modern medicine to a conspicuous degree. Modern medicine unapologetically approaches human aliments from a "treat-the-symptoms" protocol using primarily synthetic pharmacology. This is not to say, for example, that a drug prescribed to treat an infection of the digestive tract is ill conceived, but rather that this approach fails to determine what caused the infection in the first place, and whether there exists a plausible nutritional or life style factor that might prevent recurrence. This bigheaded approach birthed itself out of the scientific renaissance of the industrial revolution that extended itself well into the 21st Century, and it epitomizes the Western mindset. The human intellect was embraced as a far superior species than anything nature could contrive on its own. Unfortunately, the era of scientific enlightenment flushed thousands of years of natural pharmacology down the drain. Good for us that many of the "backward" nations, particularly in the Far East and Asia, and even some heretics in Western medicine, held on to ancient approaches to healing. This is broadly embodied in the field of natural medicine, where the least harmful and most effective conventional approaches are combined with holistic and natural medicine. The conflict between the two is substantial. The heretics integrate modern medicine into their practice but give natural healing a more prominent seat at the table of healing, while the modernists' predominately treat natural medicine with disdain. In contrast to pharmacologically driven modern medicine, natural medicine seeks to treat the overall wellness of the patient in regard to nutrition, life style choices, eating habits, digestion, stress, toxicity, etc., rather than treat the symptoms of a health condition with drugs. This is not to say that symptoms of some diseases may require a drug intervention at some point, especially with emergency or acute conditions. An Integrative doctor tries to combine the best of both worlds and only uses pharmacology and surgery when no other options are available.

In regard to preventing digestive diseases and their progression to cancer, natural medicine would argue that pharmacological approaches are helpful but they never cure the underlying cause.

Although there can be many factors that cause a digestive disorder or disease, such as toxins, allergies, bacteria, viruses, parasites, heredity, etc., natural medicine contends that the biggest factor of them all is a combination of poor nutrition and eating habits and poor life style choices. Before we look at key factors of digestive conditions, let's first review the organs that make up the digestive system:

Digestive System
1. Mouth (Oral)
2. Throat (Pharynx)
3. Salivary Glands
4. Esophagus
5. Stomach
6. Kidney
7. Liver
8. Pancreas
9. Gall Bladder
10. Small Intestine
11. Large Intestine
12. Rectum
13. Anus

All of these organs are susceptible to all sorts of diseases, including cancer. Other than some very rare cancers, these organs produce some of the most aggressive and dangerous cancers. In point of fact, four out of the five cancers with a five-year survival rate below 30 percent come from this group, namely pancreas, liver, esophageal, and stomach cancer. Lung cancer is the only other cancer with such a low survival rate. Brain and Ovarian cancer are not far behind.

The foods, drinks, and other substances we consume have a tremendous impact on the health of these organs. For example, smoking and drinking are key factors in oral, throat, esophageal, kidney, liver, pancreas, stomach, and colon cancer. They are also a causative factor in non-digestive diseases, such as lung and breast cancer. Another example is excessive consumption of sugar, which can damage the pancreas and cause diabetes. Excessive sugar consumption also leads to obesity, which is a well-documented factor in multiple cancers. Even though the larynx, which is the windpipe and voice box, is treated by a specialist other than a gastroenterologist, chronic acid reflux is a causative factor in laryngeal cancer, just like it is for esophageal cancer.[2]

According to the National Cancer Institutes SEER Fact Sheets there are over 380,000 new cases of digestive cancers each year. Digestive related cancers also cause more than 165,00 deaths each year.

The American Gastroenterological Association (AGA) claims that many aliments, including cancer, are associated with a poorly functioning digestive system. Good digestive health is principally a matter of appropriate nutrient absorption, and the ability to move food and waste products efficiently through the digestive tract. With this in mind, it makes sense that the first organs to be affected by poor diet and harmful lifestyle habits are the organs associated with the digestive system.

When these organs are under toxic stress it affects the entire body. This is why many naturopathic doctors and researchers claim that the key to good health lies in a properly functioning digestive system; in other words, a good gut.

Getting back to chronic acid reflux, its progression to cancer is something few people are aware of. Over 40 percent of people in the United States experience acid reflux at least once a month.[3] This means that if there are two people in a household, then there is a good chance that one has a chronic reflux condition and doesn't know it. They get used to the symptoms and learn to accept it as a normal part of life, when in fact it isn't. Additionally, 60 to 70 million people have some sort of digestive disease.[4]

These diseases are frequently masked by a number of common symptoms that people learn to live with so they never bring this to the attention of a doctor. These symptoms include stomach cramps, nausea, vomiting, bloating, fatigue, excessive flatulence, constipation, diarrhea, and abdominal pain, to name a few.[5] Even if they do see a doctor, digestive diseases are frequently misdiagnosed unless the symptoms progress to something severe.

I think you get the point. We are what we eat. If the digestive system is not working properly it can wreak havoc systemically.

DEMOGRAPHICS OF ACID REFLUX

As far as age goes, acid reflux is a progressive digestive disorder that gets worse as we age. It is normally not diagnosed until it becomes a chronic digestive disease, usually when someone is in their 40's or 50's.

Even though acid reflux is not common in young adults, it is surprisingly common in newborn infants and even small children. The symptoms for infants and small children are different than with older children and adults, and more difficult to diagnose because of the lack of ability of the infant and small child to communicate clearly. The good news is that most infants and small children seem to heal from acid reflux as they get older and do not require any serious medical intervention.[6] Weaning the child off the mother's milk too early is one of the suspected causes.

In regard to ethnicity, the incidence of acid reflux is highest in North America and Europe, but not far behind are certain areas of central Asia from Iran to India and China, and certain areas in southern Africa and in lower South America. Asian nations generally have the lowest rates of acid reflux. Up to 40 percent of the Western populations including Russia, experience some form of acid reflux on a monthly basis; and up to 50 percent of those have a chronic condition of weekly symptoms. The United States has the highest incidence among the Western nations.[7]

Of note, not only do Americans have the highest incidence of acid reflux but they also spend more money than anyone else on medications to treat this disease. Some of the more popular over the counter drugs other than Tums are Nexium, Prilosec and Zantac.

The problem with over the counter drugs is that you might end up like me, self-medicating underneath the radar screen, without the supervision of a doctor. Why is this bad? You will most likely end up putting a Band-Aid on the problem for years while your disease quietly progresses in the background unbeknownst to you. If you think these drugs fix the problem you are in for a rude awakening.

In 2013, the United States spent $13 billion on over the counter and prescription anti-acid medications.[8] This is 15 percent more then what is spent on coffee, $11 billion annually, and a little less than what is spent on chocolate, $16 billion.[9] It is rather ironic, but both coffee and chocolate are frequently sited as causative agents in heartburn, with a number of surveys voting chocolate as the worst offender of them all.[10]

SYMPTOMS OF ACID REFLUX

When I started researching acid reflux I was familiar with heartburn but informationally anemic in regard to Gastroesophageal Reflux Disease (GERD), commonly referred to as acid reflux. Chronic reflux and a number of other symptoms associated with GERD are the result of the lower esophageal sphincter (LES) not working properly. The LES is located at the lower end of the esophagus and remains closed except to allow food and water to pass into the stomach, or gets a signal to burp or vomit. If the LES relaxes inappropriately, acid can seep into the esophagus all the way up to the pharynx (throat), larynx (windpipe, voice box), and nasal airway, especially if lying down. It can even seep into the lungs. Unfortunately, most people like me get used to living with it and it becomes a normal part of life.

For instance, many with acid reflux experience only mild symptoms and get accustomed to living with any discomfort by taking over the counter acid indigestion drugs. These medications can easily mask something more serious. The symptoms get worse over a prolonged period and the seriousness of their condition typically goes unnoticed.[11] This is where the danger begins. If misdiagnosed, the repercussions can become irreversible and require very serious medical intervention. Even though there are many symptoms associated with this disease, most people have little knowledge of, or regard for the seriousness of the progression of something much worse.[12] This is exactly what happened to me.

Symptoms of chronic acid reflux include heartburn, pain in the upper abdominal region as well as the back, chest pain, nausea, difficulty swallowing, regurgitation of food up into the throat, vomiting, hoarseness, laryngitis, dysphagia (difficulty swallowing) chronic cough, dry cough, wheezing, sore throat, asthma, postnasal drip, chronic bronchitis, recurrent pneumonia, difficulty swallowing, bad breath, excessive belching and stained teeth.[13]

The one symptom I did not see mentioned very often during my research was chronic burping, something I had a huge problem with. I dismissed the acid reflux as a normal consequence of an injurious affair with spicy foods. What I was ignorant of is that spicy foods were not the problem. There was a much bigger problem lurking in the shadows, a damaged digestive system.

CAUSES OF ACID REFLUX

Poor Diet and Digestion

According to the American Gastroenterological Association (AGA) chronic acid reflux is primarily the consequence of a poorly functioning digestive system. In particular, good digestive health is principally a matter of appropriate nutrient absorption, ability to move food and waste products efficiently through the digestive tract, efficient immune function and a balanced community of microorganisms in the gut.

A balanced diet is critical to all of these important functions. It is not simply a matter of ingesting too much spicy food or chocolate. A digestive system that is not working properly may have other symptoms beyond those associated with acid reflux, and include frequent rumbling in the stomach, nausea, vomiting, bloating, excessive flatulence, constipation, diarrhea, and abdominal pain to name a few.[14] A poorly functioning digestive system causes further problems beyond the digestive track, because of poor absorption of nutrients, and absorption of too many toxins, all at the expense of the body's organs and immune system. Many naturopathic health experts are adamant that numerous illnesses of the body originate in a poorly functioning gut. The presence of chronic acid reflux is a clear sign of poor digestion, poor absorption and poor expulsion. Simply put, diet and eating habits are the primary factors in a broken digestive system, and a broken digestive system is the fundamental cause of chronic acid reflux.

Are there other factors that exacerbate this condition? Yes. They include, obesity and smoking, but the most serious one of them all is an anatomical condition called a hiatal hernia. Less common factors are sited as responses to certain prescription and over the counter medications, heredity, and exercising too soon after eating.

Obesity

According to the National Institute of Health and the American Gastroenterological Association numerous clinical studies identify obesity as a prominent factor in acid reflux. Extra weight in the stomach area instigates upward pressure on the LES muscle causing it to relax.

Americans have one of the highest rates of obesity in the world, at 33 percent. No wonder we also have the highest incidence of acid reflux in the world. It should not be surprising, but the United States culture is the king of fast foods, sugary foods and drinks, and processed foods full of preservatives, sodium, and other additives. Much to our chagrin, the "McDonaldization" of American culture has been exported to numerous other nations, much to their detriment. In contrast to America's highly processed, sugary and chemically infused diets, nations with low obesity rates, such as central Africa, India and Asia, depend heavily on raw fruits and vegetables grown in their back yard or locally.[15] It's time to return to backyard gardens and fresh fruits and vegetables.

Smoking

Another contributing factor in acid reflux that goes beyond poor diet and eating habits is smoking. An extensive study conducted on how smoking affects the LES muscle revealed surprising results. This study demonstrated certain chemicals in smoke cause the esophageal sphincter muscle to relax permitting stomach acid to seep into the esophagus.[16] In addition to obesity and smoking, there remains another factor instrumental in acid reflux, called a hiatal hernia, which will be examined next.

Hiatal Hernia

A hiatal hernia is an anatomical condition whereby the LES and upper muscle of the stomach relax and a small portion of the stomach pushes itself past the diaphragm into the lower area of the lung. It may stay there permanently or it can slide temporarily in and out of the chest cavity when the esophageal muscle expands and contracts during swallowing. Over ninety percent of hiatal hernias are in this category, called a sliding hiatal hernia, the one I fall into. Hiatal Hernia's present one of the most serious risk factors for chronic seepage of stomach acid into the esophagus, resulting in esophageal and laryngopharyngeal injuries and cancer.

The second type is called a para-esophageal hernia, and is much less common. In this type of hiatal hernia the gastro-esophageal junction stays below the diaphragm and part of the stomach slides up into the chest cavity. This type of hernia can result in serious complications that might require surgery.[17]

I remember Doctor R. telling me, "A hiatal hernia is not dangerous in itself, and it can be hereditary, or something acquired through obesity, pregnancy, smoking, trauma, or other factors. Many people have a Hiatal Hernia but do not have GERD, but everyone, like yourself who has GERD usually has a Hiatal Hernia. Hiatal Hernia's are fairly common and many people don't even know they have one. In most cases they can tolerate it their entire life without any trouble."

I asked Doctor R., "Is there a surgical procedure to correct a sliding hiatal hernia?" He said, "Yes there is but there is no evidence to show that correcting a hiatal hernia will correct GERD, and surgery may even make matters worse."

I also asked Dr. R. about a novel procedure that surgically implants an elastic-like band around the lower esophageal muscle to help it close. He quickly dismissed the idea and said, "In your situation there's no guarantee that it can fix things and the risks associated with it aren't worth it." At this point I realized that there is no easy fix to this complex digestive disorder.

As far as gender goes men have a much higher rate of hiatal hernia's then women, 3 to 1. It made me wonder why? Pregnancy is a known causative factor in hiatal hernia's, which seemed to contradict the fact that men have a higher incidence of hiatal hernia than women. Medical literature on this question is not clear.

When I was young I participated in a lot of physical contact sports, did a lot of weight training and also had a number of manual labor jobs that required extremely strenuous physical activity. In this regard, most women don't perform the same strenuous activities that men do, and I suspect this may be why men have a higher incidence of hiatal hernias. Moreover, esophageal cancer is also much more prevalent in men than women, indicating a strong correlation between hiatal hernias and esophageal cancer. Some experts suggest other factors might also be at work in the development of a hiatal hernia, which include prolonged vomiting from drug or alcohol abuse, eating disorders, and possibly violent coughing from Chronic Obstructive Pulmonary Disease (COPD) or other severe respiratory disorders.

Another contributing factor to acid reflux, according to naturopathic medicine, and is not commonly found in traditional gastrointestinal medical literature, is Inter Abdominal Pressure (IAP) Reflux. Let's take a closer look at this next.

A Paradox: Inter Abdominal Pressure (IAP) Reflux

One of the most fascinating things I came across while studying acid reflux is a medical concept called IAP Reflux because it speaks directly to my condition. It contradicts views of traditional Gastroenterology and is rather controversial. I was introduced to this concept by my naturopathic Chiropractor, Doctor T., and this led me to do additional research. It is widely referenced in a number of alternative medicine blogs on the Internet as a primary causative factor in acid reflux.

Doctor Eric Berg, a nationally known Chiropractor who specializes in natural and alternative medicine to help people lose weight, discusses what he believes can cause severe heart burn in a short video called "The Heartburn Myth." In this video Doctor Berg claims that acid reflux is primarily the result of the stomach not producing enough acid, and that Irritable Bowl Syndrome (IBS) and other leaky gut disorders are caused by under production of acid, not over production. He treats his patients by getting them off of anti-acid medications and replaces them at least temporarily with acid producing pills. He also puts them on a more holistic diet that avoids sugar, refined starches, bad oils and processed foods.[18] He asserts that some patients have had positive results within two days of taking acid producing pills. Is he on to something? Let's listen to an expert in another field.

Doctor Norm Robillard, a microbiologist, backs up the low stomach acid concept in his book "Heartburn Cured: The Low Carb Miracle". Doctor Robillard asserts that conventional medicine has had it all wrong in regard to the over production of acid in the stomach being the root cause of GERD. He is convinced the use of acid reducing medications do not address the root cause and in fact will make matters worse, especially in long term use. However, he doesn't refute the role a hiatal hernia, obesity or smoking play in acid reflux by causing the LES to relax. He also argues that excessive sugar and carbohydrate intake depletes stomach acid to the point that little remains to help digest meats and plant based foods. He also contends that excessive sugars and starches cause an overgrowth of stomach bacteria, which in turn produce an over abundance of hydrogen as a byproduct. Excessive hydrogen gas in the stomach puts upward pressure on the LES causing it to relax. Doctor Robillard goes on to conclude that excessive hydrogen production in the gut produces increased Inter Abdominal Pressure on stomach acids to reflux into the esophagus. His book proposes a low carb diet that a number of people claim worked for them.[19]

Those who support this concept also warn that mixing starches and meat together is a bad idea because the meat can go undigested. I experimented with this by eating a steak with French fries, versus eating a stake with vegetables. The difference was black and white. I got indigestion when I ate the steak with fries, but not when I ate the steak with vegetables. What I learned is that my stomach cannot handle mixing concentrated proteins and heavy starches, but it handles concentrated proteins with vegetables wonderfully.

The IAP Reflux concept is even more compelling when I consider my personal experience. In the months leading up to my health crisis I experienced an excessive amount of belching. I literally burped every time I ate something. It became so bad that I even burped after taking a drink of water. One day Kelly brought it to my attention and said, "Joe, what's going on with you, you seem to be burping all day long, even when you're drinking water?" I had no idea what was causing it.

After Doctor R. got me pointed in the right direction I started a daily burp-log to track any progress. Shockingly, I was burping 30 to 40 times a day. About two weeks after changing my diet and eating habits, the burping dropped off to single digits, and at the four to five week point it was completely gone. After I radically changed my diet to one high in raw vegetables and fruit, moderate in complex plant based carbohydrates, and low in fish and animal protein, my acid reflux disappeared. I also cut out spicy food, reduced coffee to one cup a day, and stopped mixing animal protein with starches. I was able to slowly wean myself off the PPI in about three to four weeks. The diet I changed to is called an alkaline diet, which is discussed in more detail in Chapter 5.

Another interesting piece of information that supports the low stomach acid concept is the use of apple cider vinegar to reduce acid reflux. There are a number of home remedy web sites on the Internet that claim apple cider vinegar cures acid reflux. Many of these web sites seem to repeat what others are saying with no scientific evidence to support their claims. They would be better served if they referenced IAP and the clinical experience of Doctor Robillard in this area, because it strongly supports their claims. I know several people who use apple cider vinegar daily and claim it reduces their acid reflux and helps their digestive system. The only thing I can conclude is that if Doctor Berg and Doctor Robillard are correct, then for at least some people, apple cider vinegar reduces their acid reflux.

So what shall we make of all this information? First, there is a strong argument reinforced by clinical medical experience that supports under production of stomach acid as a contributing factor to acid reflux. Second, taking some form of acid, such as medically prescribed pills or apple cider vinegar may help certain people mitigate acid reflux. Third, there is no proof that taking supplements to support stomach acid production will correct the ill effects of poor diet and eating habits, smoking, obesity, and a sliding hiatal hernia, not to mention stress. The bottom line is chronic acid reflux is a complex problem that requires a multi-faceted treatment approach.

ACID REFLUX DISORDERS AND DISEASES

Damage to the Esophagus

When acid reflux goes untreated, it can lead to a number of serious disorders beyond heartburn and discomfort. Chronic exposure to acid will cause necrosis of the esophageal epithelium, which is the mucosal layer of cells that line the esophagus. This condition is called erosive esophagitis. Once cells in the lining of the esophagus become inflamed it may cause strictures, which is a narrowing of the esophagus and may cause difficulty swallowing (dysphagia). Inflammation is a well-known breeding ground for disease because reduced circulation causes reduced oxygen circulation and reduced immune function. Erosive esophagitis may also result in ulcers and bleeding.

Bleeding occurs in about 10 percent of those with erosive esophagitis. If minor bleeding goes undiagnosed for a prolonged period, it may cause iron deficiency, severe fatigue, anemia, and may even require blood transfusions.[20] If bleeding is heavy it may cause vomiting. In this instance the blood would be more reddish than black in color. When blood passes through the stomach and intestines its color is pitch black. Doctors usually put patients on PPIs for at least six to 8 weeks to help bring the inflammation down and help the body heal the affected areas. These disorders can only be accurately diagnosed through endoscopic evaluation.

Laryngopharyngeal Reflux (LPR)

LPR is an acid reflux related disease that is little known. LPR is also referred to as extra-esophageal reflux disease (EERD), because stomach acid works its way past the upper esophagus into the throat, and even the sinuses. It can also find its way into the larynx and even the lungs when we breathe. It is frequently misdiagnosed and has a strong link to laryngopharyngeal cancer. Let's take a look at the anatomy of the pharynx and larynx before going further.

The pharynx is the medical term for throat, which connects the mouth to the larynx and the esophagus. The larynx is the medical term for a short tube that connects the throat to the windpipe and is located in front of the esophagus. The larynx has a small flap covering it to block food from entering when we swallow. It only opens when we breathe. The larynx, in effect, creates a temporary passageway for air to move in and out of the lungs. It also contains the voice box, which is responsible for producing the sounds required for speaking.

Symptoms of LPR are very similar to GERD, but are more commonly identified by a persistent cough, earaches, sore throat, difficulty swallowing, hoarseness, asthma and laryngitis. Many of these symptoms are shared with the common cold, allergies and asthma, causing LPR to be frequently misdiagnosed. This is why LPR is called the silent acid reflux disease.[21] Professional vocalists are in a higher risk category just from the fact they may otherwise assume the symptoms are a consequence of a tired voice, and not LPR. The lining of the larynx is much more susceptible to being damaged by stomach acids than the esophagus or throat, and this makes LPR a dangerous path to cancer.[21]

The progression of LPR to cancer is further amplified if the patient has a history of smoking or excessive alcohol use, which are contributing factors in squamous cell esophageal cancer. Very few people are aware of how serious of a condition it is, or that it is widely misdiagnosed. If it goes undetected it can progress to laryngopharyngeal cancer.[22] Anyone who has a long history of symptoms mentioned above should be evaluated by an expert in this field as soon as possible.

Progression to Barrett's Esophagus (BE)

Barrett's Esophagus is a condition in which chronic acid reflux causes irreversible abnormalities in the lining of the esophagus. Barrett's is a precursor condition to a more advanced precancerous condition, called dysplasia, and also esophageal cancer.

In Barrett's the normal cellular structure of the lining of the esophagus is changed into a premalignant state. Normal cells in the epithelial lining of the esophagus, known as squamous mucosa, are whitish in color. When Barrett's Esophagus is present, cells will take on a pinkish-salmon color because their DNA mutated into an abnormal form of columnar epithelium cells, which are intestinal-type cells found in the lining of the stomach. It is believed that cells in the lining of the esophagus go into a sort of self-preservation mode after

30

prolonged exposure to acid and attempt to transform themselves into more resilient stomach cells. Although the primary risk factor for Barrett's is chronic acid reflux, many people have Barrett's Esophagus without little or no symptoms of acid reflux. Heredity or genetic make-up is also a risk factor for those who might get Barrett's Esophagus. If you have a close family member or a friend who has chronic acid reflux, please encourage them to see a Gastro Doctor as soon as possible.

Although many experience classic acid reflux symptoms there is a significant group of people who experience very few symptoms, if any. In one study, 25 percent of the Barrett's patients had never experienced any [significant] symptoms of GERD.[23] Some of them however, experienced mild symptoms, such as colds, asthma, allergies or laryngitis. Most people are dreadfully unaware of the symptoms of GERD and that the only accurate way to determine if it has progressed to Barrett's Esophagus is through endoscopic examination.

Moreover, the prevalence of Barrett's in the general population is not well understood. Estimates range in the low single digits. This is due to the lack of using upper endoscopies as preventive medicine. Japan does preventive upper endoscopies along with colonoscopies. This might explain why incidence of deaths from esophageal cancer is much lower in Japan than the U.S.

Is there any thing we can do to prevent Barrett's Esophagus? The simple answer is yes, if we have the self-discipline to change our diet, eating habits and life style. Interestingly, some studies indicate drinking moderate amounts of wine may help reduce acid reflux and BE. In a study done in the 1990's, one control group drank a glass of wine a day while another group did not drink any wine. Those that drank wine showed a reduced risk of Barrett's compared to those that didn't drink any wine. In a more extensive study done between 2002 to 2005, 953 men and women drank one or more glasses of red or white wine a day and had a 56 percent reduced rate of BE as compared to those who didn't drink any wine.[24] I am a little guarded with these studies because there are a lot of other variables at work in acid reflux. Wine in fact may agitate acid reflux. Wine can also be terribly addictive, so please be careful.

The prevalence of Barrett's in those who have GERD is also not well understood. You may have GERD for years but not have

Barrett's, or you might have Barrett's with only minor symptoms of GERD. In general, 10 to 15 percent of those who suffer from GERD also have Barrett's Esophagus.[25] Some suggest the average time of onset from GERD to Barrett's is around 10 to 15 years.[26]

One study indicated patients with Barrett's are 30 to 60 times more likely to get esophageal cancer than the general population.[27] Barrett's patients who smoke are twice as likely to develop esophageal cancer than Barrett's patients who do not smoke.[28] Still, it is important to point out that only a small percentage of those who have Barrett's will ultimately progress to esophageal cancer.

Barrett's is not only a serious disease it is very difficult to cure. "Studies have shown that none of the medications used to treat gastroesophageal reflux disease (GERD) . . . reverse Barrett's Esophagus."[29] A recent study of almost 10,000 patients in Denmark found that long-term use of PPI's with endoscopic surveillance to treat Barrett's, presented a significant increase in the risk of adenocarcinoma or high-grade dysplasia.[30] I would never discount the possibility of PPI's being a curative factor in some cases, but most research indicates otherwise. So be careful putting your trust in pills. Eating your way out of this is difficult, but it is the safest and smartest thing to do.

Barrett's is not only difficult to cure it is difficult to diagnose. A 2014 study published in Medscape highlighted the need for more accurate diagnosis of Barrett's Esophagus. The context of this study and its findings might explain why some patients believe they were cured from Barrett's using PPI's. In this study researchers attempted to determine why there is such a wide range of prevalence of Barrett's reported by Gastroenterologists, anywhere from 1 percent to 25 percent. The average is typically sited as 12 percent. A group of doctor's reevaluated 130 patients previously diagnosed with Barrett's and discovered that 32 percent were falsely diagnosed. They stated that the margin for error in analyzing short-segment Barrett's is the crux of the problem because it is located at the Gastroesophageal Junction (GEJ). Their findings called for better definition of the GEJ when taking biopsies. They further pointed out, "The insurability issues, cost, and psychological impact associated with an incorrect diagnosis of Barrett's are considerable, and these should be avoided."[31]

In recent years, advanced endoscopic surgery options that were previously reserved for high-grade dysplasia, the final stage prior to cancer, are now being used on Barrett's patients. In one study, 136 Barrett's patients were given radiofrequency ablation, which uses a high-frequency alternating current over an endoscopic probe to burn the damaged cells away. The risk of progression to high-grade dysplasia or cancer was reduced from 26.5 percent to 1.5 percent.[32] These are significant findings that prove the value of ablative surgery. Other ablative techniques include electrocoagulation (electrical heat), argon plasma coagulation (laser heat), photodynamic therapy (PDT - laser heat), and cryotherapy (freezing). As it is for all types of surgery, ablative surgery has its own set of side effects that require close consultation with your doctor before moving forward.

Progression to Dysplasia

In the final stage of progression to cancer, abnormal cells in Barrett's mutate into an advanced precancerous stage called dysplasia. Like Barrett's, dysplasia requires analysis of biopsied tissue for diagnosis. Dysplasia is like Barrett's in that it is not reversible and can only be cured by surgery. Patient's with low-grade dysplasia are put on close endoscopic surveillance and will most likely receive ablative surgery. Patient's diagnosed with high-grade dysplasia require some type of ablative surgery or an esophagectomy, which is a radical surgery that completely removes the precancerous portion of the esophagus, and a portion of the stomach.

Progression to Esophageal Cancer

There are two types of esophageal cancer, squamous cell and adenocarcinoma. Adenocarcinoma is less prevalent than squamous cell, but it is a faster growing cancer. Adenocarcinoma forms in secretion glands in the lining of the esophagus as a tumor, in the lower or mid areas of the esophagus, and sometimes extends into the stomach. Squamous cell esophageal cancer forms as flat lesions in the mid or upper area of the esophagus, throat or larynx. In its earliest stage adenocarcinoma can be treated with surgery alone, beyond that it requires a multi-modality approach of chemotherapy, radiation therapy and surgery. In contrast, squamous cell carcinoma is frequently treated by radiation alone in its earliest stages, but more advanced stages may require chemotherapy and surgery. According to the National Cancer Institute, esophageal cancer has a 5-year average survival rate of only 17 percent. If caught in the earliest stage it has a 5-year survival of about 40 percent. If caught in a later stage, 5-year survival falls to 3 to 5 percent.[33] If it's metastatic, then survival is less than 2 percent.

Chronic acid reflux, Barrett's Esophagus and dysplasia are all risk factors for esophageal cancer. Other risk factors are male gender, over 50, obesity, smoking, alcohol abuse and a hiatal hernia.

Esophageal cancer makes up about 1 percent of all cancers diagnosed in the United States and accounts for 2.6 percent of all cancer deaths.[34] The disproportionate death rate makes it a very dangerous cancer. Men are 3 to 4 times more likely to get it than women. African Americans and whites [including Hispanics], have about the same incidence of the disease.[35]

The incidence of squamous cell carcinoma has dramatically dropped over the last 30 years; but for adenocarcinoma it has increased by 500 percent. It is considered the fastest growing cancer in the United States.[36] This same phenomenon is occurring in other Western nations too. Experts are not sure why esophageal adenocarcinoma is growing at such an alarming rate in so many countries, other than to say it is all diet and life style related.

Surprisingly, there are areas of the world that have far higher rates of esophageal cancer than Western nations. These regions include South and East Africa, South America and an area extending from the Caucasus Mountains in Central Asia to Iran, India and east to China. These regions have an incidence of esophageal cancer up to 20 times greater than Western nations. In some of these regions esophageal cancer kills more people than any other type of cancer. Experts are perplexed as to why. Some studies suggest that scolding hot drinks, such as tea, may be one of the factors that cause such a high rate of esophageal disease. One study done in Iran showed that those who pride themselves for drinking the hottest tea had an 8 times greater incidence of squamous cell cancer.[37] It appears there is a competitive game being played by males in Iran who challenge each other to see who can drink the hottest tea, something akin to many males in the United States do in regard to eating the hottest peppers.

Chronic acid reflux is a progressive disease that has a very strong link to esophageal cancer. What makes chronic acid reflux even more dangerous is that it is frequently misdiagnosed as a common ailment such as a cold, asthma or allergies. Misdiagnosing symptoms or ignoring symptoms can be a deadly mistake. Western medicine has not adopted preventive upper endoscopies for esophageal diseases. Therefore, it is up to us to become informed on the dangers of this disease; and then get our loved ones in for an upper endoscopy.

Of Note

Sociological studies indicate women spend a lot more time educating themselves on health issues than men do. Men also tend to have a bad habit of ignoring warning flags related to their health and typically avoid going to a doctor if at all possible. We also suffer from not wanting to take time off from work for health related issues. Our pride gets in the way because we want to prove to everyone how tough and indispensible we are. So, wives, daughters, sisters, and mothers, please do not let your husbands, fathers, brothers and sons put off a visit to the doctor any longer if they are suffering from any type of chronic digestive discomfort. Do not wait another day. His life may ultimately depend upon your insistence.

Notes

1. Johnson, David A., MD. "The Dreaded Diagnosis of Larynopha-ryngeal Reflux Disease", http://www.medscape.com/viewarticle/778052# (accessed April 9, 2015, 1).
2. Stat Cancer Fact Sheets. http://www. http://seer.cancer.gov/ stat facts/ (accessed October 20, 2016)
3. "Racial and Geographic Issues in Gastroesophageal Reflux Dis ease", American Journal of Gastroenterology, 2008;103(11):2669-2680, http://www. Medscape.com/viewarticle/584071 (accessed January 5, 2015, 1-4).
4. "Digestive Disease Statistics for the United States," National Insti-tute of Diabetes and Digestive and Kidney Diseases. https://www.niddk.nih.gov/health-information/health-statistics/Pages/digestive-diseases-statistics-for-the-united-states.aspx (accessed October 20, 2016)
5. "Understanding Heartburn and Reflux Disease", American Gastroen-terological Association, http://www.gastro.org/patient-center/digestive-conditions/heartburn-gerd (accessed April 17, 2015, 2)

CHAPTER 3

How To Manage Acid Reflux

Every body continues in its state of rest, or of uniform motion in
a straight line unless it is compelled to change that state
by forces impressed upon it. —Isaac Newton

One of Isaac Newton's law's of physics states that if a body is at rest, or is set in motion, it will remain in that state unless some other force acts upon it. A serious health condition that is ignored, or otherwise poorly attended, will not get better unless some other force is applied to it. Chronic acid reflux is one such poorly attended health issue, particularly in most men. Men downplay health issues and they typically put a visit to the doctor off until the condition has become acute. They also tend to neglect to follow the doctor's orders. Ignoring chronic acid reflux is a very dangerous game to play. Let's look at an example.

We already learned that prolonged use of proton pump inhibitors (PPI) increases the risk of getting cancer because they only address the symptoms not the disease. I had a coworker named David that this happened to. David was on PPI's for over 10 years, believing that there was no risk of it progressing to cancer. In his mind, he was doing exactly what his doctor told him to do. This gave him a sense of comfort, like it does for all of us—if we can't trust our doctor, then whom else can we trust? But there was one thing David failed to do, and that is to schedule an upper endoscopy at the five-year point. He simply got carried away with the distractions of life, probably thinking that since he didn't have the symptoms of acid reflux anymore then why worry. This was a huge mistake. At his 10-year endoscopy they discovered a Stage 3 tumor that penetrated the muscle and outer layer of the esophageal wall and invaded two or more lymph nodes. This was devastating news because the lymph node involvement causes a Stage 3 tumor to have as poor a prognosis as a Stage 4. What David didn't know is that recent studies of long-term use of PPI's indicate that one's risk of getting cancer increases the longer he or she is on the drugs. This happens because the drugs mask the symptoms, giving the patient a false sense of security.

These drugs are so powerful in suppressing acid production that they change the chemistry of the stomach and inhibit proper digestion of food and absorption of nutrients. They come with all kinds of unpleasant side effects too. For instance, many patients end up with erosive esophagitis after taking PPI's. Others experience an increase in heartburn and other symptoms when they cease taking these drugs, called acid rebound, which means that their reflux becomes worse than it was before they started the medication. These drugs may provide a short-term benefit, but prolonged usage is typically detrimental.

Are there any actions we can take, other than over-the-counter and prescription drugs, to manage acid reflux? Yes, they consist of a number of diet and life style changes. Can you do these things as a complement to taking drugs? Yes. The best approach is to wean our self off the drugs gradually while implementing some new habits.

The next section describes 10 eating and life style changes that are recommended by numerous Gastroenterologists and health professionals. All of them can help manage chronic acid reflux and play a significant role in helping cure it, to the point of weaning ourselves off of acid reflux medications.

10 TIPS TO MANAGE ACID REFLUX
1. Quit Smoking.
2. Drink Alcohol In Moderation.
3. Lose Weight.
4. Identify Trigger Foods And Change Diet.
5. Elevate Your Head In Bed.
6. Do Not Lie Down After Eating.
7. Eat Smaller Meals.
8. Chew Food Slower.
9. Evaluate Medication Triggers.
10. Reduce Stress.

1. <u>Quit Smoking</u>: Smoking is a well-known factor in lung and other cancers and it is also associated with acid reflux. A number of studies discovered that certain chemicals in smoke are linked to esophageal disease. Harmful chemicals produced by the combustion of tobacco are absorbed into the lungs and circulated throughout the body by means of the cardio vascular system. Surprisingly, a number of these chemicals can cause the muscle at the lower esophagus to relax allowing acid seepage into the esophagus. Barrett's Esophagus patients who smoke are twice as likely to develop esophageal cancer than Barrett's patients who do not smoke.[1] Smoking is a tough habit to break, but if living longer is important, then kicking the habit is crucial. Millions have kicked the habit and you can do it too!

2. <u>Lose Weight</u>: Obesity is a major causative factor in acid reflux and also many types of cancers. The American Society of Clinical Oncology (ASCO) states that next to smoking, obesity is the highest causative factor in cancer of the breast (postmenopausal), colon, pancreas, endometrium, kidney and esophagus. Specifically, one out of three cancer deaths is related to obesity.[2] Obesity is defined by the National Institute of Health as a body mass index (BMI) of 30 or higher. Those who are not obese but are over weight have a BMI between 25 and 30. Being overweight but not obese does not mean you are in the clear as far as risk factors go for cancer. Numerous studies indicate excessive weight is a primary instigator of chronic inflammation, which is a proven breeding ground for cancer.

ASCO also points out that the risk of cancer is directly proportional to the level of excessive weight we carry. This means that even a small decrease in weight produces a positive effect on reducing the risk of cancer.

In regard to acid reflux, we have already learned that excessive weight puts pressure on the lower esophageal muscle and causes it to relax, allowing gastric acid to seep into the esophagus. Wearing tight belts and skin-tight clothing compounds this problem further, so consider loosening your clothing a little.

The best countermeasures against excessive weight are eating better foods, changing eating habits and exercising daily. Food is very addictive, and many of us should consider enlisting some professional help from nutritionists, counselors, or trainers to stay on the narrow path to a leaner body. Seek outside help if you are unable to research your weight loss goal.

One of the greatest barriers to successfully losing weight is trying to change too many things at the same time. Most people are too aggressive in their initial goal; they fall short, get frustrated and then give up. Try to change one or two things at a time, and give yourself a reasonable time frame. Changing bad habits requires persistence, patience and time.

3. <u>Drink Alcohol In Moderation</u>: Alcohol, like tobacco, is a causative factor in numerous cancers. Many studies show a strong link between alcohol and cancers of the oral cavity, pharynx, larynx, and esophagus, and also cancers of the stomach, colon, rectum, liver, female breast, and ovaries.[3] As far as type of cancer goes, alcohol is much more of a factor in squamous cell carcinoma than adenocarcinoma of the esophagus, pharynx and larynx.

It is important to understand that alcohol may not only trigger acid reflux but also trigger an upset stomach, regurgitation and other digestive disorders. Drinking alcohol right before bed, particularly after a late evening meal, is a bad idea, because it can trigger stomach acid to seep into the esophagus, throat and even the lungs while you sleep.

4. <u>Identify Trigger Foods</u>: There are certain foods that trigger acid reflux. These foods are different for each person so it is important to spend time evaluating the things that trigger your indigestion. Nutritionists name the top culprits as spicy foods, chocolate, fried or fatty foods, coffee, tea, alcohol, carbonated drinks, tomato based foods, citrus foods and drinks, excessive sugar intake, and dairy products. Selectively take yourself off one item for at least three weeks and see if you notice a difference.

Although poor eating habits and life style choices are contributors to acid reflux, the biggest factor is most likely a highly acidic diet. Experts stress the importance of replacing sugars, starches, fatty foods and sugary drinks with raw fruit and vegetables, good oils, fruit juices, lean proteins and filtered water. When I changed to a more alkaline diet it literally changed my life. An alkaline diet will be discussed in more detail in Chapter 5.

5. <u>Elevate Your Head In Bed</u>: Anyone who has chronic acid reflux needs to elevate their head when they go to bed. Actually your torso

needs to be slightly elevated too. If you have a hiatal hernia it is even more imperative to elevate the head, because stomach acid can seep into the esophagus, throat and lungs while you sleep. If you've ever woken up in the middle of the night and felt burning in your throat, tasted stomach acid in your mouth, or a persistent cough, you have a serious acid reflux problem. It can also cause a dry cough, chronic bronchitis, sinusitis, and laryngitis. Gastroenterologists recommend that the head and upper torso be elevated at least 6 to 8 inches.

6. <u>Do Not Lie Down After Eating</u>: Doctors recommend not lying down less than three hours following a meal. Going to bed with a full stomach is a bad idea if you have chronic acid reflux, because it greatly increases the risk of stomach acid and undigested food seeping into the esophagus, throat and larynx. If you are overweight, the extra pressure on a full stomach will exacerbate the problem. This was one of my worst habits to break. I became used to eating meals or snacks late at night because of long workdays and lots of travel. It's much better to eat early meals and learn to fast the rest of the evening before going to bed.

7. <u>Eat Smaller Meals</u>: There are numerous benefits to eating five to six small meals a day instead of three large ones. First, it will allow the body to better digest the meal and empty the stomach sooner. This alone should bring about a noticeable reduction in heartburn and other symptoms. Second, it will help the body maintain a steadier blood sugar level throughout the day. Third, it will support increased metabolism and thereby burn more calories during the day and help reduce weight. Eating smaller meals not only reduces acid reflux but also plays a vital role in maintaining a comfortable weight.

8. <u>Chew Food Slower</u>: Take more time to chew your food. I think we all know someone in our family who sits down to a meal and has his plate polished off before the rest of us can place our napkin on our lap. Inhaling our food is very disruptive to our digestive system. Besides, no one wants to watch a tornado fly through the kitchen. Pausing between bites will go a long way in helping the digestive system function properly and reduce heartburn.

Some recommend chewing each bite 8 to 12 times before swallowing, and then take a pause every now and then by laying the fork down. Taking time to chew our food slower makes the meal more pleasant, aides our digestive system, and it will reduce the effects of acid reflux.

9. Evaluate Medication Triggers: Believe it or not, many over-the-counter and prescription drugs trigger acid reflux. Taking too many herbal supplements and vitamins can do this too. According to an article on Livingstrong.com, the following is a list of drugs that were clinically proven to cause acid reflux.[4]

1) Calcium Channel Blockers: Used to treat high blood pressure or hypertension, and include Amlodipine, Nifedipine and Diltiazem. These drugs can cause the lower esophageal muscle to relax.

2) Anticholinergic Agents: Commonly used to treat irritable bowl syndrome or chronic diarrhea, and include Benztropine, Ditropan and Scopolamine. These drugs slow down digestion and may cause the lower esophagus muscle to relax, resulting in acid seepage into the esophagus.

3) Tricyclic Antidepressants: Used to treat depression. They may weaken the lower esophageal muscle causing it to open.

4) Others: Iron supplements, Dopamine, Fosamax and Actonel, which are osteoporosis drugs, and Atenolol, Toprolol XL and Propranolol, which are beta blockers for high blood pressure.

Every medication and supplement should be evaluated independently for affect. If you take a number of vitamins and natural supplement it is a good strategy to split them up throughout the day and take them with meals. Taking them all at once is a prescription for heartburn.

Another caution is to not take pills right before bedtime. Undigested pills can reflux back into the esophagus. This is especially damaging if the pills are swallowed without water while lying on your back. Parts of the pill may breakup on the way down, get stuck in the esophagus and damage the lining of the esophagus while you sleep. Some experts believe this may accelerate more serious conditions, such as esophagitis [and ulcers].[5] It is safer to take all medications at least one to two hours prior to bedtime and to always elevate the head and upper torso slightly after lying down.

10. Reduce Stress: Have you ever come home after a difficult day at work and are confronted with kids fighting, a broken washing machine,

and a large auto repair bill as you frantically try to prepare dinner? Then without any planning whatsoever you eat too much dinner, or perhaps eat one chocolate chip cookie and then devour half the box, or start drinking a well intended one to two glasses of wine, but end up emptying the bottle. Or maybe you smoke a pack of cigarettes a day. All of these behaviors provide temporary emotional relieve, don't they? We all indulge our flesh at some point in our life as a form of self-medication, and before you know it, we are enslaved to some unhealthy eating or drinking habits. Long-term stress from work or family situations, or traumatic life experiences is a root cause of poor eating habits and addictions.

If you are in a stressful job, one where you feel like you are unfairly scrutinized and cannot do anything right, and you are always being asked to do one more thing, then it is time for a change. Being trapped in a toxic job is like being stuck in the nine circles of Dante's Inferno. Please do something that I was slow in doing, and that is get out of that job as fast as a snowball melts in hell. If you refuse to get off the emotional roller coaster, the emotional trauma will push your health off a cliff some day and you will be diagnosed with cancer or some other disease sooner then you ever imagined.

I recently read about a testimony given by a life long Cardiologist who reflected on what he believes is the major cause of heart attacks in men. He stated that men who never learned how to cry carried around a tremendous amount of pain in their heart. And because of this, he concluded, "They are the ones with the highest risk of dying from a heart attack." Sometimes the simplest cause and effect relationships in life are the most compelling. His professional assessment reinforced other things I studied on how diseases of the body are sometimes a consequence of profound trauma to the heart and soul, specifically physical and psychological diseases, perpetuated by negative attitudes and emotions about self or others.

If you have acid reflux, Barrett's Esophagus or cancer, it is absolutely critical you come up with a permanent plan to rid your life of excessive stress. Please do not do what I did and push your self through something that is emotionally intolerable for too long. Doing nothing about debilitating stress is a recipe for digestive disaster. So take control of your life and make reducing stress as important an item as any other we've discussed. Your life depends on it.

SUMMARY

This chapter described 10 eating and lifestyle tips that will build a solid bridge over the treacherous waters of chronic acid reflux. All of them are common recommendations given by Gastroenterologists and other health care professionals that can help manage chronic acid reflux and even play a large role in curing it. To paraphrase Isaac Newton, "a body in motion remains in motion unless acted upon by another force." Chronic acid reflux will never change unless an effort is made to change the bad habits that created it.

Life style and eating habits take time to change. Most of us have a lot of failures on the road to success, so do not let frustration rule over your mind and emotions. Be persistent but also patient with yourself. Some experts say it takes about three days to get traction on changing a bad habit, about three weeks to gain a sense of power over it, and about three months to conquer it. Reward yourself when you have success. Make changes incrementally. Climbing a hill requires one step at a time. The most important thing to remember is to never give up. Commit yourself to be the healthiest person you know, and it will happen!

CHAPTER 4

Inflammation and Cancer

Joint pain, bloating and foggy thoughts are not imagined symptoms, they're the result of improper diet. Make eliminations. Start with wheat, then dairy, then sugar. These are the most inflammatory foods.
—Nancy S. Mure, Ph.D.

H ave you ever rolled out of bed in the morning feeling sluggish and bloated like one of those cartoon-character balloons in a Macy's Thanksgiving Day Parade? I have. My fingers would sometimes swell up like little sausages and my ankles would morph into cankles. However, those days are long gone since radically changing my diet. The chronic inflammation is under control. So what's all the fuss about?

Inflammation is a well-known causative factor in cancer due to impaired circulation and the resulting accumulation of DNA altering toxins. Inflammation reduces the body's ability to move red and white blood cells into and out of an inflamed area, which reduces the body's ability to promote healthy cell growth, healing, and the removal of pathogens. Chronic inflammation is bad. Most do not understand this, that inflammation is a precursor to numerous maladies of the body, especially cancer. Long standing inflammation is also closely associated with chronic conditions such as diabetes, arthritis and obesity. According to the National Cancer Institute, "Over time chronic inflammation can cause DNA damage and lead to cancer."[1] Moreover, "Recent data has expanded the concept that inflammation is a critical component of tumor progression. Many cancers arise from sites of infection, chronic irritation and inflammation."[2] The public remains terribly uninformed on the perils of chronic inflammation.

Millions of people walk the earth each day with absolutely no clue as to why they can't lose weight, even though they hardly eat anything. This is especially true for millions who have their thyroid tested and the test comes back negative for underactive thyroid. Their doctors give them a clean bill of health because their blood work looks good. Patients continue to trudge along stupefied as to what is going on with their body. Thus, this chapter will educate patients on some of the most prominent food related causes of systemic inflammation. It will not cover everything, but focus primarily on food allergies. Specifically, this Chapter will not discuss a number of allergies that may occur from toxins in the environment, such as harmful chemicals in women's health and beauty products, carpets and building materials, electromagnetic and radio frequency fields, pollens, second hand smoke, and long-term use of prescription drugs. Americans are also exposed to pollutants being carried over the ocean by upper wind currents from poorly filtered industrial plants in China, including dirty coal-fired plants.

Accordingly, how do you know if you have an allergy to something? You can get tested by an Allergist, or cut the suspected offending substance out for a period of time and then go back on it to see if you notice any difference. A number of experts recommend that we should abstain from the suspected allergen for at least three weeks before going back on it.

Two of the main offenders, gluten and dairy, are a good place to start. If I eat a couple of servings of wheat-based pasta noodles with loads of cheese on it, and garlic bread, preceded by a cheese and cracker afternoon snack, by the next day, my nose gets runny, I sneeze a lot, my fingers swell up, and my stomach feels bloated. I also typically gain about three to four pounds and become baffled as to how it happened. What I didn't know was that my immune system goes into a tizzy when my intestine experiences gluten and dairy. My body starts producing lots of histamines and I experience an allergic reaction. Just as I got used to living with chronic acid reflux, I got used to living with chronic inflammation, in large part because I didn't understand all of the symptoms, nor did I understand that in both instances they are precursors to cancer. I cannot help but wonder how much better my health might have been, if I had not spent the last 30 years eating wheat and dairy products every day.

It's time to learn some fascinating things about common foods people are allergic to. Are you ready? Let's get started.

Common Inflammatory Triggers

1. Gluten
2. Dairy Products
3. Chemicals In The Food Supply
4. Bad Oils
5. Coffee
6. Sugar
7. Nightshade Plants
8. Stress
9. Chronic Inflammatory and Autoimmune Diseases

Gluten

So what is gluten? The highest concentration of gluten is found in wheat, barley and rye. It is a protein that does not digest well in humans. Gluten consists of large chain protein molecules that are not easily broken down by hydrochloric acid in the stomach. Consequently, they enter the small intestine undigested and too big to be absorbed. The small intestine is lined with villi, which are thin octopus like tentacles that absorb digested food, such as proteins, fat, carbohydrates, fiber and micronutrients. Gluten can get stuck in the villi and cause an inflammatory response that starts in the intestine and spills over to the rest of the body. It can also inhibit the absorption of critical micronutrients.

According to the National Institute of Health (NIH), the biggest health risk of gluten is the development of Celiac Disease. Celiac Disease is an autoimmune disease in which the body attacks its own digestive tract tissue. Only a very small percentage of people will test positive for Celiac Disease. It is loosely associated with heredity. It comes with serious digestive problems like diarrhea, constipation, bloating, inflammation, fatigue, headaches, skin rashes and even things like insomnia, mental fog, depression, and nerve problems in extremities and other areas of the body. Malabsorption of nutrients can also cause a host of other problems, such as anemia, osteoporosis and stunted growth in children.

Anyone who thinks that they might have a potential for Celiac should see a Doctor immediately to get tested for it. Celiac Disease can present with very few symptoms so be careful ignoring mild symptoms, especially if you have a digestive disease such as GERD, Irritable Bowl Syndrome (IBS) or Leaky Gut Syndrome.

One may not have a serious bowel disease yet still be intolerant to gluten. There is no test for gluten sensitivity. It is a matter of being in tune with your body and removing all sources of gluten out of your diet for about three weeks to see if you notice any improvements, and then going back on it for a day or two to see how you respond. Make sure when you go back on it, to eat a lot of it to see if you can illicit a response.

After taking myself off of gluten for only a week, I noticed an improved energy level and a reduction in inflammation throughout my body.

Everyone who has a digestive disorder needs to evaluate his or her own level of sensitivity to gluten and make adjustments as needed. There are oodles of gluten free flours available nowadays, so no one has to give up an occasional bread or pasta.

Dairy Products

Dairy products are a group of foods that most people believe are an important part of a well balanced diet, because they contain high amounts of protein and other nutrients critical for the development of strong bones, stout teeth and a healthy body. As a kid growing up, dairy products, especially milk, were an essential component of the food pyramid we learned in school. At one time or another, who hasn't seen the Drink Milk billboards along the highway, or TV commercials with prominent athletes sporting a milk mustache? Even though dairy products are nutritious, you might be surprised to learn that they may not be as beneficial to our health as previously believed. Some might say this is "udderly" ridiculous—so why don't we take a closer look?

First, dairy products are criticized because there is a strong connection between diets high in saturated fats and heart disease. Second, cow's milk is not a good substitute for a mother's breast milk. The American Academy of Pediatrics (AAP) states that cow's milk does not provide enough Vitamin E, Iron, or fatty acids. An infant's digestive system cannot handle the high levels of protein, sodium and potassium. Surprising as it may sound, it is difficult for a baby to digest cow's milk. Third, studies show 66 percent of the world population is genetically unable to properly digest milk and other dairy products because of a digestive condition called Lactose Intolerance. Over 90 percent of adults in some East Asian communities are lactose intolerant.[7] So, what is lactose intolerance and how do we deal with it?

Most humans lose the enzyme that breaks down lactose sometime during childhood; yet many of us try to eat dairy our entire lives not understanding the consequences of being lactose intolerant. Lactose intolerance can cause indigestion, stomach cramps, nausea, constipation, excessive mucous production in the sinuses, bloating, excessive flatulence, inflammation in general, and is a contributing factor to Irritable Bowl Syndrome–IBS.[8] I had to stop drinking milk when I was about 17 years old because it gave me an upset stomach. What about fermented dairy products? Like others who cannot tolerate milk, I can tolerate fermented milk products much better, such as low moisture cheese, like cheddar, which is very low in lactose. This is because the bacteria in the fermentation process produce enzymes that break down most of the lactose. A wonderful replacement for cow's milk is Almond or Coconut milk.

One of the most intimidating qualities of cow's milk is that it contains very high concentrations of a protein called Casein, which has been clinically proven to promote the growth of cancer, especially breast cancer. This is explored in more detail in Chapter 7.

If you cannot tolerate dairy products, then it is much healthier to avoid them and instead consume healthy substitute products, like Almond and Coconut milk, and non-dairy ice cream. If we have acid reflux—or other digestive disorders—or we are battling cancer—or we have chronic inflammation—or for that matter, any disease at all, we should cut diary products entirely out of our diet.

Chemicals In The Food Supply

The average American consumes an amazing amount of chemicals in their diet each year. Some of the more common ones are pesticides in non-organic foods, dyes, taste enhancers, color enhancers, emulsifiers, iodized salt, artificial sweeteners, industrial detergents used in the cleaning of food processing equipment, and plastics in the packaging.

These chemicals can accumulate in the body over time and can be extremely inflammatory.

For instance, fake ice cream, and frozen tasty treats that the Ice Cream man sells to our kids, are typically loaded with these bad chemicals, particularly all kinds of harmful dyes—yet few parents know this. So the next time you hear the inviting melody of the ice cream truck meandering through the neighborhood, please read the label before purchasing any treats. If the ingredients contain words you've never seen before, or you have no idea what they are, then it might be prudent to do a little research before consuming the product. There are all kinds of imitation ice creams in the supermarkets nowadays that are organic and consist of coconut milk, which taste fairly close to the real deal. Amy's Organic and SO Delicious ice creams are two examples.

There is one preservative that gets an honorable mention because it is extraordinarily inflammatory for many. The winner is: monosodium glutamate (MSG). As the story goes, MSG was imported to the United States from Japan following World War II, because American soldiers got hold of some K-rations belonging to Japanese soldiers. They discovered that compared to the otherwise distasteful and cheap American grunt food, the Japanese rations were exceptionally tasty—and I might add, addicting too. American's discovered that the succulence of the Japanese food was due to MSG, which acted as both a preservative and taste enhancer. Unfortunately, many of us blow up like a watermelon after eating a hearty dose of MSG impregnated foods, especially over an extended period of time. I became so allergic to it I would blow up after eating just one meal at an Asian buffet. I was also addicted to a number of the salty, crunchy, and spicy foods found in the snack isle at the grocery that are loaded with MSG. In retrospect, my epiphany on MSG solved the mystery as to why I was so addicted to Ramen soup in college—it's the MSG dumb-dumb! Asian restaurants got a bad rap with the widespread use of MSG in their food years ago, but many consumers wised up and are only eating at restaurants that advertise that they are MSG free. By the way, too much MSG can produce a terribly addictive response in the brain, something that too much sugar can do too.

Another example of a very inflammatory group of chemicals in our food supply is pesticides. They sneak into our body mostly through fresh fruits and vegetables. Traces of them can also show up in highly processed foods. Until the American farming industry was challenged with the organic food movement several decades ago, we really did not have much of a choice other than to grow our own produce organically in the backyard. Now it seems like you can find an organic option on many restaurants menus and also in most grocery stores. Let's take a look at salt next.

My take on salt is that if the body is fed natural sea salt, it is easy for the body to purge. The offending salt that causes water retention is—you guessed it, Iodized salt. A number of experts claim that too much Iodized salt is inflammatory because it has been chemically modified in a way that inhibits the body's ability to purge it efficiently. However, Iodine is important for thyroid function. This means that those who only use sea salt should take Iodine as a supplement, or make sure to eat foods high in Iodine, such as anything out of the ocean, including seaweed, and to a lesser extent eggs and grains. Another inflammatory substance in our diet that might surprise many is synthetic sweeteners, and includes, Splenda, Nutrasweet, saccharin and aspartame. All of these synthetic sugars can be highly inflammatory. Some studies indicate synthetic sugars may cause other types of allergic reactions in the body and should be avoided, or at least minimized.

We only covered a handful of common chemicals in our food supply that are potentially inflammatory. So be vigilant in reading labels and in finding ways to substitute chemical laden foods with more organic ones. It is a good thing that many Americans are starting to realize how harmful the processed food supply is. This is why there is a growing movement towards the consumption of more organic foods. It's time to start weaning chemicals out of our diet for good.

Bad Oils

For several decades, hydrogenated oils, or trans fats, ruled the shopping carts of most Americans because they were cheaper, had a longer shelf life and tasted similar to butter. They also have a higher melting point, which makes them more suitable for cooking than butter. On the other hand, trans fats are synthetically produced, placing them squarely in the corner of fake oil. Margarine, Crisco and all deep-fried cooking oils were trans fats when I grew up. By the 1990's scientists figured out, much to the chagrin of the FDA, that trans fats had some serious health issues associated with them. They cause LDL, the bad cholesterol to go up, and HDL, the good cholesterol to go down. They discovered a shocking increase in coronary heart disease when they examined the period trans fats were a staple of the American diet. So the food industry decided the gig was up and it was time to introduce cheap plant based oils into the American diet. They introduced mostly Omega 6's, which are a host of inexpensive to produce vegetable oils, including soybean, corn, cottonseed, grape seed, peanut, sunflower, canola and safflower oils. You can still buy margarine and Crisco, but they contain no trans fats. However, some of the cheaper brands still contain small portions of trans fats to extend shelf life.

The problem with these oils is that they dominate the oil we consume at the expense of Omega 3's, which are highly concentrated in fish and Flaxseed oil. Omega 6's are highly inflammatory if they are not balanced in a 2 to 1 ratio with Omega 3's. So what about olive oil? Olive oil is mostly monounsaturated fat, with high amounts of Omega 9, and is the most heart healthy of the bunch. It also has an excellent ratio of Omega 6 to Omega 3's, although it can burn easily when used for cooking. Some might ask, why am I not promoting canola oil? Canola oil is a very popular cooking oil because it has a 2:1 proportion of Omega 6 to Omega 3 fatty acids. Well, have you ever pondered what a canola is . . . ? There is no such thing as a canola. It comes from rapeseed, which is a genetically modified plant that undergoes highly industrialized processing. Olive and coconut oil are much better options for cooking, but with olive oil, you have to cook things a little slower. Another option for cooking is butter. I frequently mix equal parts of butter and olive oil for cooking. Even though butter is high in saturated fat, it is a short chain fatty acid and is easily digested.

Coffee

Coffee is one of those foods that many people have an almost romantic like relationship with—or one might say, a pronounced emotional attachment to. For sure, it's addictive qualities are world renowned, and flaunted by those under its spell as a sort of badge of honor. It also sends out a wonderful aroma. Coffee might also win the award, if there was any such award, of saving more people from being fired for being late to work than perhaps anything else. It stimulates the cardiovascular, respiratory and nervous system. In the morning it can make us feel like we got our groove on. It also has a large audience of fans who swear by it to remedy a hangover. And let's not forget all of those coffee lovers who made it through the night shift at work, or did an all nighter to study for an exam or complete a project. Some might even consider coffee to be man's best friend—next to a dog of course.

All of the good things aside, coffee is extremely acidic and can fuel the flames of acid reflux and other digestive disorders. Caffeine is also very addictive. It affects the brain in a mildly similar manner as cocaine, amphetamines and heroin, according to some experts. For those going through cancer treatment, coffee is a big no-no, because chemo and radiation place a huge acidic burden on the body. Some studies indicate that the consumption of over four cups of coffee per day may lead to premature death, and two cups per day may lead to urinary incontinence in men as they age.[3] Moreover, coffee can cause anxiety, nervousness, insomnia, dehydration, constipation, and even migraine headaches in some people. In contrast, the National Coffee Association claims coffee contains antioxidants, which are good for a healthy heart and provide additional anticancer support. The NIH conducted an extensive study on coffee with over 440,000 coffee drinkers. It found that those who drank caffeinated coffee had a 20 percent reduced risk of getting melanoma. In comparison, Decaffeinated coffee drinkers had no anticancer benefit.[4] Other studies indicate caffeinated coffee provides reduced risk of Cirrhosis, Type II Diabetes and Tinnitus.[5]

One of the most interesting things I learned about coffee was found in a study published in The American Journal of Clinical Nutrition. Researchers found that coffee can be highly inflammatory and also raise bad cholesterol. In this study roughly half of the participants drank filtered coffee and the other half drank unfiltered coffee. They discovered that as little as three ounces of filtered coffee per day increased overall cholesterol, and also increased every single inflammation marker in the body. Inflammation markers showed a linear dose-response relation to coffee consumption. This means that the rate of inflammation increased proportionally to the rate of increase in consumption. When coffee consumption reached 7 ounces per day, every inflammation marker in the body increased. In particular, C-reactive protein, a key inflammation marker in the blood increased by 30 percent, as compared to non-coffee drinkers. This study also referenced other research that indicates drinking unfiltered coffee has an even more pronounced effect on increasing cholesterol.[6] It might be a good idea for some of us who have chronic inflammation to try and wean ourselves off of coffee for a time to see if we notice a change.

Sugar

Numerous studies in animals and in humans indicate a diet high in sugar is linked to inflammation. Sugar is also linked with other serious health conditions, such as weight gain, insulin resistance, higher LDL (the bad cholesterol), and increased gut permeability. Gut permeability occurs when bacteria, toxins and undigested food particles more easily move out of the gut and into the blood stream, potentially causing increased inflammation and increased Advanced Gylcation End Products (AGE), and chronic inflammation. AGE occurs when the blood is saturated with glucose and the glucose molecules bombard healthy protein and lipid molecules to the point of causing a covalent bond without the controlling action of an enzyme. Some studies indicate that increased AGE's in the blood can cause premature aging in diabetics and oxidative stress throughout the body.

Eating foods with natural sugars in them, like fruits and vegetables, which can be high in carbohydrates, will not cause an inflammatory response unless the food is an allergen to that particular person. For example, in one study of 29 healthy people, researchers found that when each person drank only one can of soda pop per day every single person experienced a noticeable increase in inflammation markers, insulin resistance and LDL cholesterol.

Another study showed that humans who drank a single 50-gram drink of fructose experienced a spike in the C-Reactive Protein (CRP) marker after just 30 minutes, and the CRP remained elevated for over two hours. Someone eating too much bread every day can cause this same inflammatory response. Just imagine the ill effect if someone made a habit of drinking 2 to 3 sugary drinks a day year after year, or had a diet high in breads, cookies and deserts.

Keep in mind that various co-factors can weigh heavily on inflammation, in addition to excessive sugar and carbohydrate intake, such as smoking, stress, insomnia, alcohol abuse, excessive fat intake or long term use of prescription drugs.

Excessive consumption of sugar and refined carbohydrates is unfortunately an institutionalized American eating disorder. For those who wish to prevent inflammation and the degenerative diseases linked to sugar, such as diabetes and cancer, there is no other recourse than to say no to a high sugar diet.

Nightshade Plants

The Nightshade family of plants is a group of plants that have been identified as being very inflammatory for some people, but for most people they are safe to eat. For those with high inflammation markers or are struggling with arthritis, an autoimmune condition or cancer, it's worth taking a closer look at their sensitivity to Nightshades as a potential factor. Again, the only way to discover a sensitivity to one of these foods is have an allergy test done, or to cut the food out for at least three weeks to see if you experience any improvement.

Nightshades plants include:
- Tomatoes
- White potatoes
- Eggplant
- Okra
- Peppers (all types, especially the hot ones)
- Tomatillos
- Sorrel
- Gooseberries
- Ground cherries
- Pepino melons
- Tobacco
- Paprika
- Cayenne pepper
- Capsicum

A few other things to know about nightshades is that all of these plants have a substance in them called solanine, which is a glycoalkaloid poison that is toxic to humans in large doses. The amount of solanine in the fruits of nightshades is low enough for humans to eat safely. The leaves of these plants are typically high in solanine however, and should not be eaten. Also, white potatoes that are green or have green buds have much higher concentration of glycoalkaloids in them. The green portions of the potato should be cut off before consumption and the potato should not be eaten raw. There are a number of historical accounts of people who experienced acute poisoning from eating too many green potatoes or certain nightshade berries, with some going into a coma and dying within 24 hours.

Those who are sensitive to nightshades frequently report symptoms similar to gluten sensitivity, which may include serious gastrointestinal issues, inflammation, Irritable Bowl Disorder (IBD), or leaky gut.

For those struggling with inflammation and who eat nightshades on a regular basis, it might be worth their effort to get a food allergy test, or eliminate nightshades from their diet for three weeks or longer to see if their condition improves.

Stress

Although not a food, stress can be a significant factor in inflammation. As well, it can be a co-factor to a food allergy, pathogen, or other inflammation trigger. It is well documented that chronic emotional, physical or mental stress can cause a persistent inflammatory response. Couple this with other possible inflammation factors and the inflammation can become chronic and severe.

Stress causes the body to produce cortisol, which is a hormone that regulates an inflammatory response. Over time, if the trigger that caused the inflammatory response is not removed the condition becomes chronic and the immune system becomes desensitized to the cortisol. This is why those with chronic inflammation typically have higher than normal levels of cortisol in their blood. In many instances, stress is only one of several other factors that cause a chronic inflammatory response. Naturopathic medicine holds that chronic stress and inflammation, along with a bad gut and oxidative stress from a poor diet are the underlying causes of most degenerative diseases.

Let's take a look at one of the most difficult to treat degenerative diseases next, namely chronic inflammatory and autoimmune disease.

Chronic Inflammatory and Autoimmune Diseases

Chronic inflammation is believed to be either an underlying cause or a co-factor in almost every degenerative disease. Chronic inflammation and autoimmune diseases are epidemic in the United States. The difference between the two is that someone may be chronically inflamed but they do not necessarily have a disease, while autoimmune diseases may present with either local or systemic inflammation. In both cases, chronic inflammation is evident, as well as some sort of immune dysfunction. In autoimmune diseases, a serious dysfunction in the immune system triggers the body to attack normal cells and organs by mistake. Such immune system dysfunctions can be extremely debilitating and dangerous. They are also very difficult to diagnosis and treat.

We've already learned that a major risk factor in cancer is chronic inflammation, which may or may not be caused by an autoimmune disease. So what does recent research say about autoimmune diseases and cancer? Let's examine this question next.

Many recent scientific studies indicate there are a number of autoimmune diseases linked to certain types of cancer. For instance, researchers found a strong link between patients with Lupus and cancer. Lupus is 9 times more common in women than men. Research indicates that those with Lupus have twice the risk of developing pancreatic or esophageal cancer. Those with Celiac have a higher risk of non-Hodgkins Lymphoma, and those with Colitis and Crohn's are five times more likely to develop colon cancer, to name a few. In an extensive study published by the National Institute of Health, researchers concluded that multiple associations exist between a broad spectrum of Autoimmune Disease and Chronic Inflammatory conditions and cancer. They concluded that there is "a pervasive and largely positive association between 23 autoimmune and inflammatory diseases and subsequent cancer development."[9] It is worth noting that they only researched a select group of autoimmune and chronic inflammatory diseases, not all of them.

To be specific, there are more than 100 autoimmune diseases. More pervasive ones include Crohn's Disease, Celiac Disease, Lupus, Hashimoto's Thyroiditis, Psoriasis, Rheumatoid Arthritis, Type I Diabetes, Multiple Sclerosis, Fibromyalgia, Alopecia, Addison's Disease and Chronic Lyme Disease.

Conventional medicine views autoimmune disease as something that is not reversible. The first and last course of action is drugs, which are meant to target the symptoms not cure the disease, all of which have some sort of unhealthy side effects associated with them. In the most severe cases of autoimmune disease doctors have nothing more to offer than to put the patient on high dose immuno-suppressive drugs, such as antihistamines and steroids, which all come with serious side effects. In conventional medicine patients suffer a painful and never-ending journey between doctors. They Ping-Pong back and forth from one specialist to the next—never finding a cure. There is however another medical approach to treating autoimmune diseases that very few know about. Are you ready? Let's take a look at it now.

In contrast to conventional medicine, naturopathic and functional medicine approaches the autoimmune problem from a whole different angle. They look at the entire body as an integrated system and seek to use safe and natural approaches to healing. They contend that a primary contributor to most autoimmune diseases is a poorly functioning or damaged digestive system. This is not to say that other factors might be at work, such as heredity, gene mutations, parasites, viruses, bacteria, stress, lack of sleep, tobacco and alcohol abuse, or exposure to various toxins.

Although Naturopathic Doctors are well versed in treating autoimmune diseases, there exists someone more specialized in this field, called a Functional Doctor. A good example of one is Doctor Oz, who has a daily syndicated TV show on health. In a very tangible way Doctor Oz is revolutionizing western medicine by bringing a more natural approach to healing.

Functional doctors focus on treating the underlying cause of a disease not its symptoms. They zero in on things like diet, a healthy gut, the immune system, toxins in the environment, sleep, stress, and the mind-body connection to achieve a balance between a healthy body ecology and mental-emotional state. Functional doctors will point out that conventional medicine falls short because they look at a specific organ as being the problem, not the whole body as an interconnected system, and this is why they have no cure for this type of disease.

There exist substantial clinic evidence that doctors who treat autoimmune diseases with a more natural approach achieve much better outcomes than conventional medicine.

There are also many remarkable testimonies of patients who experienced a significant mitigation of their disease or a complete reversal. Some patients are even able to go completely off pharmacological intervention and back to a more normal life.

From my experience, most people have never heard of a Functional Doctor, so please get the word out to those who are suffering the crushing blows of an autoimmune disease.

Summary

Chronic inflammation is an underlying precursor for numerous diseases, particularly cancer. Yet, most people remain dreadfully unaware of the dangers of chronic inflammation. These are people that are to some degree also overweight. Be that as it may, if you intersect eating too much of an inflammatory food with an environmental allergy, you have a prescription for persistent inflammation. Short of going on a water and vegetable only fast for a couple of weeks, a person who has a significant food or other allergies is going to have difficulty losing weight no matter how hard they try. So, for those who have a difficult time losing weight, it is time to start isolating foods that are the most common perpetrators of inflammation. Try fasting from a suspected offending-food for three weeks, go back on that food for a couple of days by eating a high dose of it, and then see what happens. You will be amazed at what you might uncover. Also consider a consult with a Functional or Naturopathic doctor, especially if you have chronic inflammation or an autoimmune disease. If you are trying to prevent cancer, or its recurrence, then it's even more critical that you purge inflammation out of your body for good.

Notes

1. "Chronic Inflammation," National Cancer Institute, https://www.cancer.gov/about-cancer/causes-prevention/risk/chronic-inflammation(accessed October 20, 2016).

2. Cousins, LM, Werb, Z., "Inflammation and Cancer," Nature. 2002 Dec 19-26;420(6917):860-7 https://www.ncbi.nlm.nih.gov/pubmed/12490959 (Accessed September 30, 2015, 1-2).

3. Coffee Consumption Linked With Reduced Melanoma Risk, 21 January 2015. http://www.medicalnewstoday.com/articles/288316.php (Accessed September 30, 2015, 1-2).

4. Ibid., 1.

5. Ibid.

6. "Associations between coffee consumption and inflammatory markers in healthy persons: the ATTICA studh1'2'3', Antonis Zampelas et al. The American Journal of Clinical Nutrition, Am J Clin Nutr October 2004 vol. 80 no. 4 862-867, ajcn.nutrition.org, 1-6.

7. "Lactose Intolerance," http://ghr.nlm.nih.gov/condition/lactose-intolerance (accessed April 3, 2015, 1).

8. Ibid.

9. Alexis L. Franks and Jill E. Slansky, "Multiple Associations Between a Broad Spectrum of Autoimmune Diseases, Chronic Inflammatory Diseases And Cancer," PMCID: PMC3329285, Anticancer Res. 2012 Apr: 32(4): 1119-1136. https://www.ncbi.nlm.nih.gov/pmc/articles/PMC3349285(assessed January 15, 2018)

CHAPTER 5

Food As Medicine

Let food be thy medicine and medicine be thy food.
—Hippocrates

Have you ever watched television during primetime and noticed the types of products that we are targeted with? Tums, Tums, Tums! Acid indigestion drugs are one of the more popular commercials. Americans want quick fixes for every problem, particularly our health. What can be more convenient than fixing a health problem by popping a pill? Instant gratification is the Western modus operandi.

I watched these commercials for years and placed my trust in messages that portray these drugs as a normal part of life. Everybody gets heartburn, bloats, burps, and has burning in the throat all the time, right? Unfortunately, I clicked my heels and popped the magic pills one too many times and found myself in an emergency room with an internal bleed and an esophageal tumor—not back in Kansas. These medications masked a serious disease for many years.

The good news is that anyone can be healed from, and prevent acid reflux, and most digestive disorders, including most ailments, by simply changing their diet and lifestyle habits. Good nutrition is medicine for a myriad of ailments. The flip side to this is that poor nutrition causes the illness in the first place. Most doctors will tell us this. Just look at Type II Diabetes, a disease that people literally eat their way into. And so it is with obesity, a progenitor of all sorts of ailments including cancer. We are what we eat. So why do so many of us eat our way into bad health, but have no idea how to eat our way into good health? Perhaps we're conditioned to believe that medicine is only pills, elixirs, diagnostics, clinics and hospitals. Or, perhaps it's one big cultural cop-out. Or, maybe we simply lack knowledge on what good nutrition is. If it's the latter, then this chapter offers a delicious main dish of knowledge, right off the self-empowerment menu. It's time to serve dinner now.

So back to the earlier question: how did I cure years of chronic acid reflux with diet? I simply changed my diet to a mosaic of alkaline foods and cut the bad things out. This chapter presents research-based information that shows how critical diet is to our overall health, specifically in the context of poor digestion as one of the root antagonists. This chapter also identifies foods and substances that harm our digestive tract, damage our immune system, and provide fertile soil for cancer. But before we do this, lets look at the root cause of a broken digestive system.

CAUSES OF DIGESTIVE DISORDERS

Other then a viral, bacterial or parasitic infection, or the ingestion of something toxic, there are five underlying causes of most digestive disorders, and for that matter, most illnesses.

Nutritional Deficiencies. There are two categories of nutrition: macronutrients and micronutrients. Macronutrients are the main source of energy and consist of protein, fat, carbohydrates and fiber. Micronutrients are essential substances and consist of things like vitamins, minerals, enzymes, amino acids, essential fatty acids, and anti-oxidants. Micronutrient deficiencies can cause a whole host of illnesses. Less advanced countries typically suffer higher rates of macronutrient deficiency than Western countries. On the other hand, nutritional excess with the wrong foods can also lead to micronutrient deficiency.

Nutritional Excess. This occurs when macronutrient consumption is critically out of balance, such as a diet high in sugar and processed carbohydrates. It causes the digestive system to break down and results in excessive build up of fat. Eating too much of the wrong foods usually means we are not getting enough of the good foods. It also causes malabsorption of micronutrients leading to nutritional deficiencies and numerous degenerative diseases.

Stress. Stress is a well-known factor in numerous health issues. It negatively impacts multiple functions throughout the body, including the mind and emotions. In regard to digestive disorders, stress can cause such things as ulcers, nausea, vomiting and an upset stomach. Reducing stress is a key piece to every health puzzle.

Intestinal Dysbiosis. This occurs when intestinal bacterial colonies are damaged, resulting in poor digestion. For this to happen, the percentage of pathological bacteria is too high relative to the percentage of beneficial bacteria. Probiotics and fermented foods like yogurt and Kimchi, help restore healthy bacteria and proper absorption.

Chronic Dehydration. Many health problems, including the impairment of the operation of the body's organs, can be caused by chronic dehydration. Dehydration causes constipation, urinary incontinence, poor digestion and malabsorption of nutrients. It is not possible to flush all of the toxins and waste material out of our body each day if we are not drinking enough water.

OUT OF BALANCE DIET

If we eat too many bad foods at the expense of good foods, our diet becomes out of balance and we end up nutritionally deficient. If there is a single food that stands out more than anything else as nutritional excess in Western diets, it is sugar. The type of sugar we are talking about is highly processed white sugar that has zero micronutrient value. Confections, which are food products loaded with sugar and other ingredients, also fit into the sugar category. I exclude honey, maple syrup, molasses and Stevia because they contain both macronutrients and micronutrients. Stevia is natural plant-based sweetener. It is very low in calorie content, tastes wonderful, and is approved by the FDA as a safe substitute for sugar.

Many things taste better if there is a little sweetness added to them. This is why sugar is put into about every single product we can find on the grocery shelf, save meat, fish, and produce. Sugar substitutes that are synthetically processed are not the answer. Various studies link synthetic sugars to all sorts of health problems. Sugar-based confections frequently contain dyes, emulsifiers and preservatives to make the confections look and feel good, and prolong shelf life. Many of these added substances are also linked to cancer.

Numerous studies show the link between sugar and foods with a high glycemic index, and how these foods produce an addictive response in the brain. Foods with a high glycemic index are starchy foods like white flour, processed starch, and white potatoes. A study published in the American Journal of Nutrition examined a control group of overweight men and scientifically proved the addictive nature of sugary and starchy foods. They found that sugar and foods with a high glycemic index, compared to low sugar and low glycemic foods, trigger a strong hunger and craving response for food up to four hours after eating these foods, in every single subject in the control group.[1] The foods this study is speaking to are breads, noodles, white rice, white potatoes, flour based snacks, and all types of desserts. Like sugar, highly processed starchy foods have very little, if any, micronutrient value. The result is an out of balance diet, weight gain and nutritional deficiencies. Unfortunately, highly processed starchy foods are relatively inexpensive, enticing low and middle-income families to spend disproportionate amounts of their income on them, as compared to fresh fruits and vegetables.

Children are also terribly susceptible to food addictions and many become hooked on sugary foods at a young age. Their brains are not able to rationalize the concept of how something that tastes so good could possibly be bad for them. The food industry understands this fact and spends a lot of money targeting children. The food industry also has a lock on our politicians. They are not required to warn the public with labels that expose the addictiveness of sugar. American parents and our overindulgent culture are not much help either. We have pretty much institutionalized Halloween, Christmas, and Easter as sugar centric holidays, where each generation of parents who fall under the spell of sugar wonderland, pass it on to their children. And so it goes.

According to the Centers for Disease Control and Prevention, 1 out of 5 children aged 3 to 19 are obese, 70 percent of Americans are overweight, over 80 million are pre-diabetic, and over 20 million have Type II Diabetes, because of having too many glucose producing foods in their diet.

Sugar and highly glycemic foods produce health problems that go beyond obesity and diabetes. They place tremendous strain on the body's ability to maintain a healthy pH level. Lets examine this topic more closely next.

HEALTHY BODY pH CHEMISTRY

The human body has a complex system of regulating the level of acidity in its fluids, organs and cell tissue. The importance of keeping acidity at an optimal level can be likened to the importance of keeping the fuel, oil, and coolant in an automobile clean. If the fuel in your car is contaminated, then your car might misfire or it might not even start. So it is with the level of acidity in our body's fluids. Too much acidity and our body's immune system starts to break down wreaking havoc everywhere.

So what causes an overly acidic body? It is a consequence of eating and drinking too many acid producing foods and drinks. Other contributing factors are long-term use of over the counter and prescription drugs, absorption of chemicals from hygiene and cosmetic products, unfiltered well or spring water that is polluted by nitrates and other toxins, and absorption of chemicals from toxic objects in our environment. Our body's filtering system can only filter out so many things each day. If it falls behind, toxins build up, acidity levels rise, and we are more susceptible to disease. Let's now look at pH and elaborate on this concept further.

The Acidity Scale: The following explains how to interpret pH.
– Acidity is measured by the concentration of hydrogen ions, referred to as potential hydrogen (pH).
– pH is measured on a scale of 0 to 14.
– A pH of 7.0 indicates neutrality and divides the scale between acids and bases.
– Numbers less than 7.0 and moving towards 0 indicate increasing acidity.
– Numbers beginning at 7.0 and moving toward 14 indicate increasing alkalinity, or base.
– Soda has a pH of around 2.5 and is extremely acidic.
– Pure water has a pH of around 7.0.
– The optimal pH in our blood is 7.35 to 7.45, slightly alkaline.
– Our body works around the clock to keep our blood pH in the above range, more so than any other area of the body. Anything even slightly

below this produces a very serious condition called acidosis, which can result in organ shut down and even death. Fluids in the rest of the body are also slightly alkaline, except for urine and stomach fluid. Advanced cancer patients are always extremely acidic because the by-product of cancer is lactic acid.

If the amount of acidity we produce in our body reaches a certain critical mass it will overload our immune system. Few of us have ever heard of the concept that the types of foods we consume not only affect our entire digestive system but also impact our body pH-chemistry. Let's next take a look at the pH of certain types of foods.

ALKALINE AND ACIDIC FOODS

Fresh vegetables, including root vegetables, are the most alkaline food group. When digested they produce an alkaline affect on the body. Nuts can range from slightly alkaline to slightly acidic, depending on the nut. Some fruits produce a highly alkaline effect on the body, such as lemons, limes, grapefruit, and oranges, but most other fruits are slightly alkaline or neutral.

When sugar is added to fruit juices it makes them produce an acidic effect. Brown rice is more neutral in pH. White rice and all types of grain-based breads are slightly acidic. Fish can be either neutral or acidic depending on the fish. Shellfish are acidic. All meats, eggs, and dairy, including butter and margarine, are acidic. Sugars, sweets, refined starches, sodas, coffee, condiments, alcoholic drinks, prescription and over-the-counter drugs, vitamin pills, plus all canned foods and microwavable foods are acidic.

See **Appendix A** for a more detailed breakdown of foods broken down by level of pH.

Naturopathic experts recommend 75 percent of our diet should be balanced towards more alkaline foods. Western diets are more likely closer to 25 percent alkaline. A number of experts believe this is one of the main reasons why we are such an unhealthy culture. Now it's time to take a look at the effect that an overly acidic diet has on the immune system, according to various experts.

Acidic Foods and the Immune System: If you don't think that highly acidic foods, such as sugar and starchy carbohydrates, have a negative affect on the immune system, then contemplate this: Have you ever noticed the number of people who get colds between Thanksgiving and New Years? Maybe like me, you are one of them. Year after year it's the worst time of year for illness. Why? Conventional medical theory claims cold weather brings peak virus season and people cluster together indoors in multiple venues and spread viruses to each other.[2] We might as well add the fact that people do not wash their hands enough either.

Here's another theory to contemplate—a contributing factor if you will. Imagine what most people do as far as eating habits during holidays. When we cluster together indoors, don't we consume generous quantities of deep-fat fried foods, cookies, pies and desserts, and imbibe excessive amounts of sugars in our sodas and other holiday drinks? The point is, excessive sugar brings our immune system down and is a big factor behind the virus peak during the holidays. Are you ready to look at some of the science that explains why sugar is detrimental to our immune system? Let's do it.

Vitamin C and the Immune System: Four decades ago, Doctor Linus Pauling, a world-renowned microbiologist, discovered the critical function Vitamin C plays in allowing white blood cells to absorb and destroy viruses and bacteria. He calculated that white blood cells require 50 times more Vitamin C than other cells in the body. If this level is not maintained the immune system is weakened.

Glucose molecules and Vitamin C have a similar cell structure. Consequently, white blood cells absorb glucose as readily as they do Vitamin C. When the concentration of glucose rises above 120, white blood cells end up absorbing too much glucose to the detriment of Vitamin C. Doctor Pauling calculated that if this situation occurs, then white blood cells would lose up to 75 percent of their capacity to absorb Vitamin C, and they would become crippled in their ability to destroy pathogens.[3] He also found that when white blood cells are saturated with glucose, it takes four to six hours before they regain their full capacity to destroy pathogens.

Doctor Pauling's research provides a key factor to help explain the excessive amounts of illness during holiday periods. This is why many health professionals recommend we load up on Vitamin C during the holiday season at the first signs of a cold.

I learned something else fascinating about the use of Vitamin C in medicine. There are a number of naturopathic doctors who recommend intravenous (IV) Vitamin C infusions as a method to bolster the immune system in people fighting cancer. The stomach can only absorb so much Vitamin C per day. Intravenous Vitamin C bypasses this constraint. Not to say that taking high doses orally does not help, it is just not as effective for cancer patients. There are varying opinions on how much oral Vitamin C to take daily to boost the immune system. Many suggest taking three grams (3,000 mg) to 10 grams per day. You know you've taken too much when your stools get loose or experience diarrhea.

Doctor Pauling is not the only one that preaches sugar avoidance. Nancy Appleton, PhD in Nutrition, reinforces Doctor Pauling's research on the damaging effects of sugar on the immune system. She wrote an excellent book on how excessive sugar is a root cause of numerous illnesses and diseases, entitled: *Suicide by Sugar: A Startling Look at Our #1 National Addiction.*[4] She does a terrific job explaining the damaging effects of sugar on the immune system and its direct link to illness and disease. This is a good book to read if you are a sugar or starchy food addict.

What then? If sugars and associated refined starches are the Big-Bad Wolf disguised as Grandma, then what food groups are best for little Red Riding Hood?

The Value of an Alkaline Diet: The American Cancer Society (ACS) recommends that every American should consume a minimum of five servings of fruits and vegetables each day. Why? These two categories of food are loaded with nutrition and highly supportive of our immune system, especially in preventing cancer. They are high in anti-oxidants, vitamins, minerals, micronutrients and substances like calcium, potassium and magnesium, which are critical for maintaining proper digestion. Even though the ACS does not expressly say it, these food groups produce a powerful alkalizing effect on the body. They are also rich in an anticancer agent called Glutathione.

Glutathione is a well-documented anticancer amino acid. It is primarily produced in the liver but requires precursor amino acids for absorption from the food we eat. The precursor amino acids are found in all types of food, including fish and meats, but are highest in fresh fruits and vegetables. Dairy products like raw milk and egg whites, and a mother's breast milk, are high in it as well. Glutathione is the most abundant intracellular sulfur-bearing antioxidant found in the human body. It serves as a significant scavenger of toxins, including pesticides, solvents and heavy metals, and blocks free radical damage to all types of cells.[5] This is one of the reasons why the ACS and many other health experts recommend we eat lots of raw fruits and vegetables.

However, this important immune system agent can be destroyed when food is cooked at high temperatures, especially when food is burned. If we choose to cook our vegetables, it is always much better to only partially cook them, thereby retaining as much of their anticancer capability as possible. Canned vegetables retain very little glutathione. The only food preservation methods that do not significantly damage glutathione or its precursor amino acids are pickling, freezing, and freeze-drying. Extensive research shows glutathione is not easily absorbed as a synthetic supplement. Injecting glutathione directly into the bloodstream is the most effective delivery method when used as an immune system booster.

Fresh fruits and vegetables earn five gold stars for being the best vitamin pill out of all the food categories and in producing the most alkalizing effect on the body. Lets next take a closer look at the biology behind the negative impact of an acidic diet.

An Acidic Diet: According to Doctor Susan E. Brown in her book, *The Acid Alkaline Food Guide*:

> Chronic acidity in the body causes the cell-to-cell process through-out our body to become impaired because oxygen and nutrient absorption are severely impaired and cells are not able to expel toxins efficiently, causing these toxins to build up at the cellular level, and frequently causes fatigue and all manner of disease.[6]

Doctor Brown and many other researchers identified this modern day disease as chronic low-grade metabolic acidosis. Throughout human history our diets were rich in fruits, vegetables, nuts, lean proteins, and healthy plant-based oils. This changed during the Industrial Revolution with the mass production of processed foods. Western diets evolved away from highly alkaline healthy diets to highly acidic and toxic ones. The introduction of sugars into every type of processed food imagined is the state of affairs of the Western food supply. One can hardly walk down an aisle in a grocery store and find an item on the shelf that does not contain some form of high fructose corn syrup, or sugar. Please keep in mind what we already learned about sugar and other foods that cause inflammation; they are precursors to cancer.

Jonathan Aviv, a renowned American Otolaryngologist (Ear, Nose and Throat Doctor) and Surgeon, authored a book about the connection of acid reflux to Esophageal and **Laryngo-Pharyngeal Reflux** (LPR) cancer, and how to cure acid reflux with an alkaline diet. This is a rather groundbreaking approach for a traditional doctor who does not profess to be a naturopath. Promoting a healthy diet as an antidote to illness is a huge departure from Western medicine, one many are glad to see.

He is not only an expert in accurately diagnosing LPR, but has fantastic success treating it with changes to diet. His success in treating LPR bears witness to his treatment approach and he is reportedly gaining a huge following among his peers.

In regard to acidity and toxins, Doctor Aviv points out some startling information. In the 1970's, the Food and Drug Administration (FDA) implemented Title 21, which approved 333 different preservatives and additives that the food manufacturing industry may use in our food to prevent spoilage. He claims that little oversight by the government became the norm, in regard to notifying the public about any harmful effects these additives might have on our health. Doctor Aviv clearly identifies these additives being purposely acidic to deliver longer shelf life.[7] Now it's time to discuss other groups of foods that should be treated with caution.

FOOD GROUPS NEEDING CAUTION

Animal Proteins: All red meats, which include any animal with a hoof, shellfish, poultry, and fish, are concentrated proteins. They have an acidic affect on the body, especially red meats. High red meat consumption comes with some serious cautions other than it being highly acidic. First, red meats contain high levels of phosphorus. When meat is digested it produces a high level of phosphoric acid in the blood. Sodas also produce high levels of phosphoric acid. Red meats inhibit the absorption of calcium in the small intestine. When phosphoric acid levels are high, the kidneys are not able to adequately expel this acid without drawing additional calcium from bones, teeth and nails. "This has a disastrous effect on bone density."[8] It can also lead to kidney stones. Meats increase the levels of sulfuric and nitric acid in the blood too, which place additional burden on the kidneys to neutralize them with minerals before they can be filtered out. Moreover, Vitamin D plays a crucial role in the body's ability to use calcium. This means a Vitamin D deficiency along with a heavy acid load on the kidneys is a prescription for Osteoporosis.[9]

As far as cancer goes, a number of studies prove excessive red meat consumption is a high risk factor for gastric, pancreatic and esophageal cancer.

It makes sense to reduce intake of red meats if battling a digestive disease or cancer, and for that matter, any sort of illness, and substitute it with more plant-based nutrition. Chapter 7 will discuss animal based proteins and cancer in much more detail. Next, lets look at another caution that goes with high meat consumption.

Highly Processed Meats: Highly processed meats, which include hams, hotdogs, lunchmeats, bacon, sausage, and smoked meats and fish, should be avoided because they contain synthetic preservatives, namely, sodium or potassium nitrates and nitrites. Nitrates and nitrites are chemical compounds used in the curing process to prevent bacteria from growing in the meat, to improve flavor, and to help retain a natural color. Nitrates are found naturally in the soil, in vegetables and dairy, and are also manufactured synthetically. Synthetic sodium nitrates are used in fertilizer, pyrotechnics, and rocket propellant. Some researchers have linked the nitrates found in red meats and processed fish, including smoked fish and meat, to stomach and esophageal cancer.

So how do nitrates increase the risk of cancer? During the digestion process, bacteria in the saliva, stomach and intestine convert nitrates to nitrites. These nitrites then bond with proteins to produce nitrosamines, which are documented carcinogens.[10] Nitrosamines are the malefactor not the nitrates. A similar chemical process is believed to occur in highly processed or smoked meat and fish. It is suspected that over saturating the meat or fish with nitrates accelerates the conversion process to nitrosamines.

The transformation to nitrosamines is also accelerated when one burns meat or fish. This is a good reason to avoid eating burned fish and meat, or at least trim the burned areas off.

The word is out on nitrosamines, and food manufacturers are

starting to provide a greater range of healthier choices on the super-market shelf. Even so, read the labels carefully before putting anything into your grocery cart.

Not to be surprised, there is plenty of literature that refutes the linkage of sodium nitrates and nitrites to cancer, claiming it to be a myth. The argument goes like this. Since we consume nitrates in vegetables all the time they must be safe to eat. I suspect this argument comes from meat industry supporters. It is an interesting argument, but I don't buy it. Why? Naturally occurring nitrates in things like celery and spinach also contain antioxidants like vitamin C, which prohibit the progression of nitrates to nitrosamines. Second, adding nitrates to processed meats and fish might saturate the meat and accelerate protein conversion to nitrosamines, when the meat otherwise would not have done so. Third, laboratory tests on animals prove that nitrates used in processed meat are carcinogenic in animal studies, yet no such tests show nitrates found in vegetables do the same. Although this subject remains controversial, it is an easy call for me—avoid consumption of highly processed or smoked meats and fish.

More On Nitrosamines: In addition to processed meats, nitrosamines are found in numerous consumer products. I do not want anyone to think nitrosamines are lurking behind every bush, but we live in a very toxic world, and there are multiple avenues for nitrosamines to enter the body. To that end, following are some common products that contain nitrosamines.

Consumer Products that Contain Nitrosamines
– Dairy products, including Nonfat Dairy Milk
– Rubber/Latex products: party balloons and condoms
– Cosmetics
– Pesticides: from commercially farmed produce.
– Well water: unfiltered well water has the potential of containing high concentrations of nitrates from inorganic fertilizers.
– Tap water: get your water tested for pesticides and other chemicals, or at least put a carbon filter on the faucet and replace it every 30 to 60 days. They cost less than 20 dollars at the hardware store and they are easy to install.
– E-Cigarettes: several brands of e-cigs have tested positive for nitrosamines.[11]
– Cigarettes

– Chewing Tobacco
– Beer

Let's take a closer look at chewing tobacco and beer. Why? Men have a much higher rate of oral, esophageal and gastric cancers than women. Men also consume chewing tobacco and beer products at a much higher rate than women. I hope men who read this will see there is something much more significant than a casual relationship to certain male lifestyle habits and cancer.

Smokeless Tobacco: Nitrosamines are found in all forms of smokeless tobacco. Smokeless tobacco is dangerous because it contains all sorts of cancer causing agents. Many who chew tobacco might argue that smokeless tobacco is much safer than smoking. But it really isn't so. Non-tobacco users probably do not know that people who dip for a long time end up swallowing the juices—it gives a better buzz. Just imagine how acidic this makes the stomach and how much injury it could cause to the mouth, throat, esophagus, stomach and the intestines. Smokeless tobacco products have a number of other carcinogens to worry about, namely benzopyrene, and polonium 210, a radioactive element found in tobacco fertilizer.[12] The National Cancer Institute warns that there are a total of 28 chemicals in smokeless tobacco proven to cause cancer. The types of cancer directly linked to smokeless tobacco are oral, esophageal and pancreatic, and it may also cause heart disease.[13]

Beer: I hate to spoil the fun further, but if you like to have a cold one with your chew, there are nitrosamines in beer, although they are not at high levels. Beer also has gluten in it. For big beer drinkers, there might be some gluten to beer belly mischief going on as well.

There was a huge scare in the late 1970's over nitrosamines in beer. Beer manufacturers went on a huge marketing campaign to deny the presence of carcinogens in their beer and the American public, for the most part, swallowed it. The FDA, to their credit, under intense lobbying from beer manufactures to deny any such claims, acknowledged nitrosamines existed in beer and set a safe limit of no more that five parts per billion (ppb). Unfortunately, the FDA did not require beer manufacturers to place a warning label on their products with tested levels of nitrosamines.[14] Beer manufacturers ultimately improved their manufacturing processes to minimize nitrosamine formation during malt kilning, and by 2006, less than one percent of all beers sampled in the U.S. exceeded the FDA's five ppb requirement.[15] Several imported beers tested by the FDA had high levels of nitrosamines in them, so it would be prudent to perform some due diligence on imported beers you drink on a regular basis.

In any case, during the media beer bash over three decades ago, WLS-TV in Chicago, Illinois, commissioned Thermo Electron Laboratory (TEL) in Waltham, Massachusetts to perform an independent study of 18 popular beers. Roberta Baskin, an investigative journalist for WLS-TV, is actually the one who initiated the independent study and broke the story. The story went on to make national headlines and was even on the Johnny Carson Show.[16] In order to make your own assessment on how much beer you should be drinking on a daily basis, provided is a list of some of the beers that were tested by TEL with their associated levels of nitro-sameness.

Domestic Beer: Nitrosamines in ppb* in 12 oz.

Stroh 2.0
Pabst 2.2
Old Style 2.5
Lowenbrau Light 2.7
Miller High Life 2.8
Olympia 3.1
Budweiser 3.3
Schlitz Lite 3.8
Michelob 5.5
Schlitz 7.7
Old Milwaukee 9.2
Erlanger 18.8
Heineken 6.9
Heineken Special Dark 23.4[17]

*Note: The FDA measurement is in parts per billion (ppb), not parts per million (ppm) as referenced by the source for this information.

Other Acidic Substances: Other acidic things we consume are medications, vitamin pills, herbal supplements, power drinks, sodas, and alcoholic beverages. All of these substances place added burden on the digestive system and produce acidity in the body. Long-term use of over the counter and prescription medications can also cause all sorts of other negative side effects on the body.

Unfiltered Water: Public tap water across the United States may meet minimum FDA standards for cleanliness, but in reality, tap water frequently contains trace amounts of metals, pesticides, industrial chemicals and detergents. Over time, the body accumulates these toxins in fat and connective tissue. Attaching a small carbon filter on the kitchen faucet is not a difficult task, and the benefits far out weigh the small cost. Some of the natural or spring water sold at grocery stores is not much better than the average tap water. Always read the labels of store bought water to make sure it is filtered.

Rules of Thumb For Mixing Food Groups: The types of foods we combine in a meal, unbeknownst to most people, affect how well we digest and absorb nutrients. For example, pairing a concentrated protein, especially a red meat, with a concentrated starch, such as a potato, is a bad idea. Why? The meat might go largely undigested. If you like your meat and potatoes, then at least take a meat related digestive enzyme with your meal. It is much better on the stomach to eat vegetables with meats, and starches with vegetables. Also, fruits digest better with vegetables and even better separately. Pineapple is a rare exception and can be eaten with meat. It contains bromelain, an enzyme that helps digest meat. Undigested food prohibits the absorption of micronutrients, potentially resulting in vitamin and mineral deficiencies. If meats go undigested, it can create a breeding ground for yeast, parasites and cancer cells in the intestines. Undigested, or putrid meat, can be a cause of foul smelling stools.[18]

General Guidelines for Mixing Food Groups
1. Eat concentrated proteins with non-starchy vegetables.
2. Eat grains and starchy vegetables, like potatoes, with non-starchy vegetables, like cucumbers and lettuce.
3. Eat fruits by themselves or only with vegetables.[19]
4. If you can't resist mixing combinations of foods that don't digest well together, take a digestive enzyme and eat smaller portions.
5. Chew each bite of food longer. Some suggest that we should chew each bite 12 to 15 times, not the standard eight times.

Summary

An unbalanced diet produces poor digestion, acid reflux, weight gain, malabsorption of nutrients, inflammation, highly acidic body ecology, and a compromised immune function. The end result is a framework for all manner of disease. However, a more alkaline diet, focused on fresh vegetables and fruit can turn many health problems around and give the body the right chemistry and nutrition to heal itself. If you are battling cancer, or trying to prevent its recurrence, than an alkaline diet is a critical element for success.

Nevertheless, making long term changes to our lifestyle, eating habits and diet can take time, so do not become frustrated with yourself if you seem like you are not making much progress. Start changing eating habits one small bite at a time, not everything at once. Reward yourself with a treat every now and then. If you backslide a little, cut yourself some slack, but then get up the next morning and recommit yourself to conquer the thing that has a chokehold over your life. If you find yourself stuck in a rut, then consider enlisting the assistance of a dietician or nutritionist, or even an exercise trainer to get you back on track. There is much greater freedom in saying no to things that are harmful to us than being in bondage to them. Refuse to quit, and you will never regret it. Break those chains and set yourself free!

Notes

1. American Journal Of Clinical Nutrition; Lennerz et al, "Effects of Dietary Glycemic Index on Brain Regions Related to Reward and Craving in Men". June 26, 2013, doi: 10.3945/ajcn.113.064113.

2. Park, Madison, "Four ways to Avoid Getting Sick During the Holiday Season". http://www.cnn.com/2010/HEALTH/12/20/sick.holidays (accessed April 24, 2015, 1).

3. "Sugar and Your Immune System," http://alternativehealth atlan ta.com/immune-system/sugar-and-your-immune-system (accessed April 24, 2015, 1-3).

4. Appleton, Nancy, PhD, "Suicide by Sugar: A Startling Look at Our #1 National Addiction," 1st ed. Garden City Park, NY: Square 1 Publishers, 2008, 1-7.

5. Murray, Michael, Dr. et all. "How to Prevent and Treat Cancer With Natural Medicine," New York, N.Y.: The Penguin Group, 2002, 31.

6. Brown, Susan E., M.D., Trivieri, Larry Jr. "The Acid Alkaline Food Guide: A Quick Reference To Foods And Their Effect On pH Levels." 2nded., Garden City Park, NY: Square One Publishers, 2013, 2.

7. Aviv, Jonathan E., MD, FACS. *Killing Me Softly From Inside: The Mysteries & Dangers Of Acid Reflux.* North Charleston, Charleston, S.C.: Create Space Independent Publishing Platform, 2012, 7.

8. Barefoot, Robert R. and Reich, Carl J., M.D. *The Calcium Factor: The Scientific Secret Of Health And Youth*, Southeastern, PA:Triad Marketing, 2002, 21.

9. Ibid, 22.

10. "Nitrosamines", Mosby's Medical Dictionary, 8th edition 2009, Elsevier. http://medical-dictionary.thefreedictionary.com/ Nitrosamines

11. "What Are The Dangers Of Nitrosamines?" http://www. electroniccigarettesale.net/what-are-the-dangers-of-nitrosamines (accessed April 23, 2015, 2).

12. "Establishing Tolerance Limits for Tobacco Specific Nitrosamines (TSNAs) in Oral Snuff under the Massachusetts Hazardous Substance Act Mg L 94". http://archive.tobacco.org/Documents/010821oraltsn. htm (accessed April 23, 2015, 2-3).

13. "Smokeless Tobacco and Cancer", http://www.cancer.gov/cancer-topics/causes-prevention/risk/tobacco/smokeless-fact-sheet (accessed April 25, 2015, 2).

14. "Nitrosamines in Beer", Posted by Bob Sink, May 10, 2007,https:// beerinfood.wordpress.com/2007/05/10/nitrosamines-in-beer (accessed April 23, 2015, 1-2).

15. Brewing Science 01/2007; 60(5/6):84-89, http://www.research gate.
net/publication/233854541/Reduction_of_Nitrosamines_in_Beer-
Review of a Success Story (accessed April 23, 2015, 1-2).
16. Baskin, Roberta, "Investigative Reporting | A Reporter's Notebook".
http://www.kosmosjournal.org/article/investigative-report-ing-a-
reporters- notebook (accessed April 23, 2015, 2).
17. Ibid., Nitrosamines in Beer, 2.
18. Food Combining: "The Little-Understood Secret To Optimal Health &
Weight Revealed". http://bodyecology.com/articles/food-combining
-optimal_health_and weight.php (accessed March 19, 2015, 2).
19. Ibid., 2-4.

CHAPTER 6

A Moment In Paradise

How many are your works, Lord! In wisdom you made them all;
the earth is full of your creatures. There is the sea, great and
wide! It teems with countless creatures living things
both large and small. —Psalm 104:24-25

Early that morning I fished the non-bathing sections of the beach and caught numerous whitefish and yellow-blue pompano's. Shortly, I would be on my way to meet up with Kelly who always preceded me to the beach on the mornings I fished. Life could not have been better. I stayed a little longer than normal that morning, because the fish were biting—probably because we were in a full moon. By now, I had been using the same lure that I had caught from the mackerel for over a month. As was my custom, I rarely kept any fish. Instead, I enjoyed the exhilarating feeling of catching them, and then letting them slowly slip out of my hands, back into the cozy womb of the ocean. Before releasing them I would hold them in my hands and admire how beautifully they were created. This made it even more difficult to let them go. But I always did. Letting something go—or so I like to imagine, always has a more satisfying feeling than keeping it. Sometimes life is like that too. At times, it is good to let go of something.

It was almost five weeks since being admitted to the hospital for an upper gastro bleed, but it seemed light years away. We enjoyed our time together too much to worry about my health, especially since the acid reflux was gone, and I was able to wean myself off the medication. I remember boasting to Kelly, "I haven't taken a Tums in over a month." This was a comfort drug I had lived with for many years but now its hook on me sank to the bottom of the sea.

As I approached the beach, the salty air and fresh breeze enticed me to draw nearer. This time I had some business to discuss and would pick a time carefully, not wanting to spoil the moment. As I reached the pathway to enter the beach, 30-foot palm trees stood guard on mounds of sand, further inviting me to enter their sanctuary. I stopped for a moment, to take it all in and give my heart and mind a moment to genuflect.

We spent the rest of the day reading, swimming, and relaxing at the beach. As the sun started its descent I knew it was time to bring up some unfinished business. I broke the silence and said, "Kelly, after I went fishing this morning I called the doctor's office to schedule the follow-up endoscopy. I should have probably called a little earlier but I didn't see the urgency in it." She said, "I'm not worried. Your biopsies were negative and you shouldn't have anything to worry about." I said, "You're right, but Doctor E. is out of the country and the earliest opening is in three weeks, which makes me a little nervous. Life seems perfect right now and I don't want anything to change that." She said, "I wouldn't worry at all. You are the healthiest I've seen you in years."

The next three weeks passed quickly, and I soon found myself waking up again on a bed in an outpatient clinic at the hospital. This time I was not able to wake up so quickly. The Doctor needed to hit me with another dose of anesthesia because he had to extend the procedure, which is never a good sign. After I woke up, the doctor had already left the recovery room, but he had debriefed Kelly. With a pale look on her face she said, "He took a large biopsy this time and needed extra time to stop the bleeding. He also tried to wake you for several minutes, but as soon as your eyes opened they shut closed. He couldn't wait any longer, so he debriefed me and moved on." He told Kelly, "The mass does not look normal. You should hope for the best but prepare for the worst. I'll put a rush on pathology and give Joe a call tomorrow with the results."

When Kelly finished debriefing me I sensed our moment in paradise had come to an end, or so it seemed—it was time to let go.

CHAPTER 7

What Do I Do Now?

You've got to be very careful if you don't know where
you're going, because you might not get there.
—Yogi Berra

The night of November 13, 2013 did not sojourn well. It was brutal and unsympathetic. Doctor E. would call me today with the results from the biopsy. I suppose I was in denial. Isn't that one of the phases everyone goes through prior to accepting an inscrutable difficulty? I remember lying there, in the shadows of the morning, in a cold sweat, contemplating my situation. I tossed and turned all night, tormented by the fear of getting cancer and what that might entail as far as changing my life forever. I contemplated the reality of death. Among my thoughts was an ill feeling that of all the days it could have been, it was the 13th. "Thirteen is supposedly an unlucky number," I thought, "but would it bear true today?" My past experience spoke otherwise. I had never had a problem with 13, even Friday the 13th. So why should my heart faint with sorrow now? Doctor E. told us to prepare for the worst. How do you prepare for being hit by a lightning bolt? I felt as if someone had just shouted at me, "Here it comes, duck!" But there was no place to duck. Do you shake your fist at heaven? Or, do you sit down and cry? My faith instructs me to accept it and make the best of whatever God has permitted in my life; something that takes super human strength to do, the type of strength I did not think I possessed. I needed something outside myself to lift me up. So, I sought after it.

I decided to get up before Kelly and seek the solitude of the beach and the ocean. Before I could squeeze myself out the door Kelly hooked me. She said, "Joe I was praying for you this morning and I was given a verse in the Bible and I believe God will heal you." I glanced back at her and said, "Thanks." I did not know what else to say. I could not bring myself to say the word cancer, nor was I ready to talk about it. I could not accept the idea that I could have cancer. Needless to say, I spent the entire day withdrawn from Kelly in quietude and reflection.

During that day I could not help but call to mind many events in my life since my youth. In particular, I recalled a number of spectacular healings I experienced—things I had not thought about for many years. It made me wonder what triggered it. Perhaps it was Kelly telling me that God would heal me, before we even had the results of the biopsy.

In one instance, when I was 16 years old, I fell like a dart, head first from a 16-foot obstacle at a Civil Air Patrol Survival camp at Hawk Mountain in Pennsylvania. The impact should have snapped my neck and killed me. But it didn't. I remember regaining consciousness with my eyes still closed, and hearing a panicked Camp Officer say, in a desperate voice, "I can't get a pulse, I think he's dead." I was glad to be alive, yet I could not feel anything in my extremities. It seemed as though I broke my neck and was paralyzed from the neck down. The hospital took three or four sets of X-rays, and each time the doctor would say, "I don't see any broken bones. Take him down for another set of pictures." Finally, they gave up. They kept telling me it was a miracle that I was still alive and that there were no broken bones. Within several hours following the x-rays, I started to regain feeling in my toes, then my fingers, and then the healing slowly migrated throughout the rest of my body until I regained movement. Every one on that floor of the hospital wanted to walk in and see the kid that survived a near fatal fall and wasn't even paralyzed. I was amazed at what happened, and could not help but spend some time simply thanking God again for His mighty healing hand. I recall thinking, "How could such a wonderful turn of events become so far from my mind for so many years? Are we innately ungrateful creatures?"

In another instance, I experienced a serious bout of mononucleosis in college. I was terribly sick for well over a year. The Epstein-Barr Virus (EBV), a member of the herpes family, causes mononucleosis. In rare cases it can progress into certain lymphomas and other cancers. At about the one and one half year point, they performed extensive blood work and took full body x-rays. My white blood cell count was through the roof and numerous lymph nodes were enlarged all over my body. I next saw a Hematologist, who suspected lymphoma, so he ordered a biopsy. I reported to the hospital for the biopsy and expected to hear bad news. As I was being prepped for surgery, the surgeon walked in, plucked my medical record from a basket attached to the wall and slowly paged through it. He walked over to me and examined the glands in my neck and then said, "I see no need to do a biopsy at this point. Your blood work looks normal and the glands in your neck are not very large."

Again, everyone was in awe at such a miraculous turnaround. However, I know what caused it—my mom's prayers. All of us have had miraculous events occur in our lives, and perhaps like me, we neglect to call them to mind except in a desperate moment. I recalled other such things that day, where I could have been terribly injured or killed but escaped calamity. They could not have come to mind at a better time. I found new strength in them. They gave me hope.

A Turning Point: It was 5:45 pm on the evening of the 13th, as I was just pulling into our parking space after being gone all day when my phone rang. Kelly was inside so I decided to take the call in the privacy of the car. I put the car into park, turned off the radio, and reached for my cell phone. An afternoon shower lightly sprinkled the windshield, while the wipers droned back and forth. As the phone continued to ring, I held it in my lap and checked the caller ID—it was Doctor E. He said, "I just visited pathology and I'm sorry, I do not have good news for you. The biopsy confirms you have adenocarcinoma at the junction of the esophagus and stomach. Time is critical because this is a fast moving cancer. I am going to order a CT scan, PET scan, and endoscopic ultrasound (EUS) immediately so that we can stage the tumor and get you into treatment as soon as possible. I will do everything I can do to help speed up the process." I asked, "How big is the tumor?" He said, "I estimate it to be about 4 cm (1.6 inches). The urgency in Doctor E.'s voice said it all. However, I needed a few moments to collect myself before I delivered the bad news to Kelly. So I sat in the car quietly, as the rain gently pattered the windshield.

I entered our apartment, walked over to Kelly and before I could finish saying, "Doctor E. called," she said, "Joe, I know you have bad news." I said, "Yes, you're right, it is not good and I'm really afraid. What do I do now?" She paused, and then said, "Can I pray over you?" It was time to claim the verse she gave me that morning.

We decided that we needed a little more information before we should start making phone calls. Then we decided it would it be beneficial to sit down and make a list of action items that needed to be done right away. This was the smartest thing we did that night. This list got us focused and organized, and became an invaluable roadmap on how to press forward. It gave us an immediate sense of empowerment after feeling so helpless.

This chapter summarizes a number of things patients can do right away that will allow them to set an anchor in a treacherous sea.

Ten Things To Do Right Away

1. Activate Your Faith, a Positive Attitude and a Support Group.
2. Set-up an Efficient Communication System.
3. Establish a Prioritized Action List.
4. Make Healing a Goal and Set it in Motion.
5. Understand Survival Rates.
6. Understand Staging.
7. Understand Treatment Options.
8. Set Up Diagnostic Tests and Transfer Medical Records.
9. Understand How Referrals and Insurance Work.
10. Chose a Cancer Treatment Center.

1. Activate Your Faith, a Positive Attitude and Support Group: After activating our faith with prayer, we tried to figure out who to notify first and what to say to them. We needed a little time to absorb the blow, so we waited a day before making any phone calls. In addition, I wanted to spend a night studying this type of cancer and its survival statistics before talking to others about it. During these early moments we also made a list of family and friends that we wanted to bring in on this. A support group is extremely important, and mine was a tremendous source of encouragement and strength throughout treatment. Kelly was of course my main line of support, but a secondary tier of others would bolster both of us.

The Mayo Clinic claims the benefits from positive thinking, among other things, may increase lifespan, provide greater resistance to the common cold, lower rates of depression and lead to better psychological and physical well being.[1] There are also a number of studies that show the impact of a positive attitude on healing. In one such study, researchers found that when faith and prayer are put into a category of meditation, there is strong scientific support proving spirituality has a positive effect on healing. This study was published by the National Center for Biotechnology Information (NCBI) under the National Institute of Health and stated the following:

> Different types of meditation have been shown to result in psychological and biological changes that are actually or potentially associated with improved health. Meditation has been found to produce a clinically significant reduction in resting as well as ambulatory blood pressure, to reduce heart rate, . . . to boost the immune response, . . . to reduce anxiety and pain and enhance self-esteem . . . .[2]

I asked one of my oncology nurses, who was a breast cancer survivor, "How important is it to have a positive attitude in the healing of cancer patients?" She replied, "In over 30 years of treating cancer patients, those with the most positive attitudes are always the ones with the best outcomes." Doctor O., my Oncologist, and every other person in the treatment center, at one time or another, stressed the importance of a positive attitude. So our faith, along with a positive attitude, and a support group, places us in a position to achieve the best possible outcome with our disease.

2. Set Up an Efficient Communication System: Next, we set-up an efficient system to communicate with everyone in our support group. One of the best ways to do this is to establish a patient website. There are a number of services that are free on the Internet. Two of the more popular ones are caringbridge.org and carepages.com. These free patient websites allow one to set up a password-protected website and send out periodic updates to everyone at once. It also allows family and friends to communicate with each other. We decided to do something different and inform them through a group email. It was simple to set-up and it worked beautifully. Kelly put together a weekly update and sent it out. Those who wished to comment could respond back to us privately or to everyone else as desired. It is easy to get overwhelmed by everything involved in fighting cancer. We simply do not have the time or emotional energy to talk to everyone on a regular basis. This is especially true as you become incapacitated with fatigue by the chemo, radiation, or surgery. Setting up an efficient communication mechanism proved to be well worth the effort.

3. <u>Establish a Prioritized Action List</u>: Some very important decisions need to be made early on in the process and numerous actions need to be taken. Experiencing panic and feeling like your life has just come unraveled is the norm. Indecision grips all of us to some extent. The best thing to do is to get organized and sit down with a pen and paper and make a simple list of things that need to get done. These are things that you can start attacking right away. It also provides a great sense of direction and control. Even greater, when a complex problem is put down on a piece of paper it doesn't seem as complex anymore. The action list allows the emotional vertigo to stabilize.

A good way to organize the action list is to prioritize each action item using the A, B, C system, where each letter represents a different degree of priority. The list becomes a living document that is easy to amend daily. You don't need to build an excel spreadsheet or put together a 10 page project plan. A simple piece of paper or notebook will work fine. Keep it simple and sweet! Once you start tackling action items, be careful not to try to do too much at once, because you can quickly feel overwhelmed again. Focus on one thing at a time. Any daily progress you make is important because it gives positive traction that pushes the locomotive down the healing track, one choo-choo at a time.

If you don't have a spouse or partner, then please find a family member or friend to sit down with to help you develop an action list. The action list will get you focused and organized. It will empower you to take charge of our treatment plan an impact your destiny. Please do not delay in getting one started.

4. <u>Make Healing a Goal and Set it in Motion</u>: When we get cancer it is very tempting to let go of everything and throw ourselves at the feet of the cancer treatment center and demand they heal us. In essence, it is tempting to detach ourselves from any responsibility we might have to be healed and assign it to the doctor. This is the wrong attitude. We can let ourselves become a victim of a tragic Shakespearian play, closed in on all sides by a villain with no chance of escape, or we can embrace the role of a protagonist and do things that resist our unpleasant circumstance. Moreover, throwing our treatment outcome entirely in the laps of our doctors and caretakers is an extraordinarily unfair thing to do to them. I sort of know what this feels like.

While teaching in private high schools early in my education career, on several occasions, a parent would come up to me and tell me how difficult their child is to handle at home, and that they expected me to fix their child. I assured them that without the parents working with me at home in a team effort, their child would not get fixed. They needed to have a bigger stake in the ground then I did. I believe most medical professionals are no different. They are purposed to do everything in their power to help us heal. Yet, they also want us to become partners with them in the healing process.

I learned something else as a teacher and coach, and in my own struggles in life that helped me take a determined stand against my disease. There is something extraordinarily powerful about setting a goal in a deliberate manner. First, the goal must come from deep within, and it must be backed by strong emotion and a good intention. In other words, put an energetic smiley-face on it. Secondly, the goal must be set in motion by some action that seeks to accomplish it. The most powerful first step we can take is to write the goal down on a piece of paper and then articulate it verbally to others around us. The thought is affirmed by writing it down, and validated by the verbal action. To put it another way, the action infuses a certain amount of kinetic energy to something that was previously motionless. This is why many teachers and coaches have students and players write down their goals at the beginning of the school year or sports season, and then have them articulate it back to their teacher or coach. Later in the school year the goal is reviewed several times to monitor progress. These simple actions demonstrate a sincere intent as well as a certain level of commitment that had not been previously present.

Additionally, tell everyone around you, including your doctors and nurses that you are determined to get completely healed. Once you start this process tell yourself, "There is no turning back. I can't quit!" You owe it to yourself, and to your family and friends to give it your best effort every single day, no matter how bad you feel, or how difficult the treatment becomes. With cancer, every single effort we make to accomplish our goal to be healed matters!

5. <u>Survival Rates:</u> Be careful evaluating survival rates, because what-ever you are staged at does not necessarily indicate what your outcome might be. Always place yourself, both mentally and emotionally, in the percentage that survives no matter how small that number might sound. If you adapt many of the things suggested in this book, then you will have a much better chance to upgrade your survival statistic, compared to having done nothing. Especially, since the remainder of

this book equips patients with numerous holistic measures they can take to substantially improve their outcome.

The five-year average survival rate for esophageal cancer, which includes both squamous cell and adenocarcinoma, is about 17 percent––not a very chirpy statistic to contemplate. This makes esophageal cancer among the worst. It is as lethal as lung and liver cancer, both with five-year survival rates of around 16 percent. I placed myself in the smallest portion of the statistic—the ones who survive—and I haven't let go. Therefore, claim a future healing, pray for it daily, and tell yourself constantly that you will be among those who survive.

6. Understand Staging: Staging is difficult to understand. It depends on a rather complex formula requiring accurate diagnostic tests and pathology reports, which are imperfect. Additionally, certain conditions in an earlier stage may place it in the survival statistic of a later stage. Initially, I estimated my tumor as no more than a Stage T3 because of its size. My guess was actually pretty close because they later staged it as a T2b, with suspected lymph node involvement. However, lymph node involvement placed it in a less optimistic prognosis. I hope you do what I did and take the time to inform yourself. It will make your doctor and nurse's job a little easier and you will have much more peace knowing what is going on.

A detailed explanation of staging is provided in **Appendix B**.

7. Understand Treatment Options: As far as treatment options go, there is essentially a one-size fits all for esophageal cancer, as it is for most other cancers. It is referred to as the Standard of Care (SOC) for that particular disease. The SOC for any disease is approved by the FDA and is strictly regulated. Doctors and nurses have virtually no say in how they are to treat cancer patients, including the types of drugs, technology, procedures and treatment options they use. Federal regulations provide the rules and regulations for the entire industry and are then promulgated to the state level for implementation. State Medical Agencies regulate the medical industry by implementing and enforcing FDA directed rules and regulations and by the issuing of licenses to practice medicine. Any significant deviation from a SOC might cause them to lose their license to practice or be hit with a lawsuit due to malpractice for not following a SOC.

Patients always have the right to seek a second opinion, or opt out of any component of treatment they disagree with. My experience was that a second opinion is nothing more than a different flavor of the same ice cream. Nevertheless, in the absence of any other options, the pressure exerted on the patient to conform becomes a do or die proposition, in the mind of the patient. In fact, on at least three occasions I tried to explain to a nurse or doctor my desire to opt out of the surgery and I was asked each time, "How bad do you want to live." It was not until much later that I discovered some alternative cancer therapies I would have pursued first, if I had known about them. This topic will be explored more in Chapter 14.

8. Set Up Diagnostic Tests and Transfer Medical Records: It is vital to get the diagnostic tests scheduled as soon as possible so that the cancer can be staged. Without this information, the cancer center will not be able to develop a detailed treatment plan. Secondly, this means all diagnostic tests and medical records used to diagnose and stage the cancer need to find their way to the cancer treatment center prior to the first appointment. Therefore, medical records go hand in hand with the importance of the diagnostic tests.

The diagnostics I needed were a CT scan, a PET scan, and an endoscopic ultrasound (EUS). All three of these diagnostics were completed within two weeks of the diagnosis. This was close to record time, thanks to the help of Doctor E. and his staff. Getting all the needed diagnostic tests completed can easily take over a month. Knowing that the cancer is growing during this time is disquieting. However, we will later explore some powerful holistic antidotes patients can safely do at home during this wait and see period. Additionally, diagnostics and appointments all require referrals from the primary care doctor to the insurance company for approval. This will be discussed in detail in the next section.

Once the treatment plan is determined, there is additional time required to schedule the chemo, radiation or surgery, and to prepare the patient for the treatments, such as surgically implanting a chemo port under the skin. The chemo port is typically inserted under the skin in the upper chest below the clavicle. The chemo port allows a catheter to be inserted into an artery in the neck, and then it is threaded to a point close to one of the heart valves. The objective is to quickly disperse the toxic drugs over the entire body, thus avoiding a harmful concentration in any particular area.

In regard to medical records, it is time-consuming and frustrating having them transmitted to the cancer center quickly. I decided to have copies transmitted and also to hand carry a copy of the diagnostics used for staging, including the most recent endoscopies, and pathology report. Besides, if you want another opinion you won't have to jump back on the medical-record hamster wheel. If records fail to show up on time, you might have to reschedule your appointment, which is the last thing you want to have happen. Hand carrying medical records greatly mitigates this risk.

The process for getting records transferred requires a signed request for transmittal by the patient at each facility he or she was seen at. I had records at seven different locations. Painfully so, they all use different forms. I hate doing administrative stuff but it's a necessary evil in this process. Getting all of these records transmitted quickly felt like a swarm of flies buzzing around my head. I had to hunt down each one patiently until it landed, and then smack it with a fly swatter to get the little bugger out of my life.

I decided to do all of the transmittal requests in person, even though some offices allow transmittals over the Internet. If you choose to order medical records over the Internet, a separate patient account with an associated logon ID and password are needed. I got exhausted thinking about doing this. I already have an umpteen number of Internet accounts, so adding seven more might have put me into the Guinness Book Of World Records. If you go in person, at least you have a point of contact and a number in case anything falls through the cracks. Be careful in filling out contact information for the office that is to receive the medical record. Mistakes such as entering an incorrect phone or fax number are easy to make. Every record that is requested for transmittal should be followed up with a phone call to the receiving doctor's office. It is easy to assume that your primary doctor or specialist is keeping track of all of your records, after each flaming hoop you jump through, but this is simply not the case. To be clear, no one else has more responsibility for your records than you do!

Getting into a treatment center quickly takes a lot of phone calls, visits and tracking. Things get overlooked and people make mistakes, so be the one driving the bus. Most administrators who handle medical records are doing the best job that they can; yet they are typically over tasked. Therefore, be patient with them. Remember, we all make mistakes, so be gracious with everyone and always give a smile and a cheerful thank you back to those helping you.

9. <u>Understand how Referrals and Insurance Work</u>: Dealing with insurance companies can be treacherous waters to swim in. It is imperative to understand how referrals and insurance work to move things along quickly and to avoid surprise medical bills. The primary doctor, or Primary Care Manger (PCM) is required to initiate a referral to the insurance company for every appointment with a specialist, diagnostic test, or procedure prior to it being approved. Once the insurance company receives a referral, it either approves or denies it. If a referral is denied, someone needs to get on top of it immediately and find out why. And that person is you!

Once you make an appointment, it is vital to understand any co-pays you might have. Do you make 20-dollar co-pay, or do you pay 20 percent of the procedure? You need to ask these questions and find good answers for them, because the insurance sharks are hungry creatures.

In one instance, a diagnostic center assured me that all I owed was the co-pay and then later sent me a bill for everything else the insurance company failed to pick up. I almost had a heart attack when I opened the bill. We had moved from Bradenton to Orlando to be near the treatment center but the bill was never forwarded to our new address. Consequently, I found out about the bill months later when a collection agency started harassing me and I discovered a negative entry on my credit report. By the way, never talk to a collection agency, because they are ruthless predators and will attempt to threaten you with huge fines and lawsuits, extorting money out of you. This is illegal, by the way. Talk to your insurance company first and find out what happened, and then deal directly with the company that billed you.

Interestingly, the way the insurance system works is that the medical center sends a retail price to the insurance company for the visit, test or procedure. By prior agreement, the insurance company only pays a contracted price. This contract price is much smaller than the retail price, typically only about 25 percent of it. The bill sent to you is the retail price and it does not reflect what your insurance company intends to pay. If you have good insurance coverage, the insurance company pays the contract price and the co-pay is predetermined, as per the insurance plan.

The moral of the story is talk to the medical center's business office and verify what you are responsible for financially, before going ahead with the test or procedure. Be advised that you may get bills in the mail after the fact. I received bills with huge additional co-pays associated with them, almost a year after completing treatment. Keep all records associated with the treatment for at least a year. Do not blindly pay a bill sent in the mail without first verifying its accuracy, because insurance companies sometimes make mistakes and there is lots of mail fraud out there. This is especially true in Florida.

Another astonishing fact is how the medical industry is biased against cash paying customers. Believe it or not, the people who do not have insurance, the poorest and most disadvantaged among us, and also small business owners who cannot afford insurance, are the only ones who pay the extreme retail rate. That's right, cash paying customers get hoodwinked. Many people who don't have the cash have to either sell their small business, cash in their 401K, sell their home, or find a non-profit organization, including the cancer treatment center to help them out. In fact, the biggest cause of bankruptcy in the United States is from earthquake-like medical bills. Some of the stories I read surrounding this problem are heartbreaking. So be vigilant with insurance.

10. <u>Choose a Cancer Treatment Center</u>: The United States has numerous cancer treatment centers throughout the country. Deciding which one to seek treatment at is a rather daunting and time consuming task. Many of these cancer centers are also world-renowned. In fact, the National Cancer Institute (NCI) designated 68 institutions as National Cancer Research Centers across the country that receive government subsidies and they are all topnotch institutions.

I looked for a center that had a well-established history of treating esophageal cancer. Look for a center with a high volume surgical center, where the doctors are experienced in your type of surgery. I started my search by asking my doctors, nurses, family and friends for recommendations. I developed a list consisting of centers in the southeastern region of the United States, which all fit my requirements. All the centers I looked at offered the standard of care treatment.

However, one center was different, the Cancer Treatment Centers of America, in Atlanta, Georgia. They offer a more integrative approach to whole body healing, using nutrition, diet, exercise, natural supplements, and spirituality. CTCA was at the top of my list because I wanted an integrated approach that included naturopathic medicine as a complement, but they were out of network.

My vetting process went as follows. I read every cancer center's website on my list along with patient testimonies and took a few notes. Then I called every one of them and spoke to an admissions representative and took a few more notes. The first thing to ask is whether they accept your insurance. The second thing to ask is the earliest date you can get an appointment. Third, determine what diagnostic tests are required for the appointment. Finally, ask all the other things that are important to you, and do not be afraid to call back with follow-up questions later, if necessary.

MD Anderson in Orlando offered me the earliest appointment, so I went with them.

Summary

Getting cancer is a devastating blow. If we let our emotions rule, they will entrap us in a perpetual cycle of anxiety, fear, and indecision. At some point we need to pick ourselves up, brush ourselves off, roll up our sleeves, and swing back with hope and determination.

It is paramount to take control of our cancer early on, by developing a plan and putting it into action. By taking control we empower ourselves as a key participant in the healing process.

Following is a summary of key things that drive a stake in the ground and allow us to take charge of our healing:

– Activate our faith. Healing starts in our attitude and faith.

– Pursue a positive attitude daily, and establish a support group.

– Set up an efficient communication system.

– Put a prioritized action list together.

– Make healing a goal and set it in motion by writing it down and then express it to every one around you.

– Take the time to understand the survival rates for your disease, how staging is performed and the treatment options. The better you educate yourself, the easier it is for you to understand what your doctor and nurses are trying to tell you.

– Mentally and emotionally place yourself in the survival statistic that is healed from cancer, no matter how small it might be.

– Set-up diagnostic tests immediately, and make sure all medical records are managed and transferred efficiently.

– Understand how to initiate and track referrals, and how insurance works. Verify how much of the bill you are responsible for prior to moving ahead with every test and procedure.

– Keep all insurance related records for at least one year.

– Take time to research a cancer treatment center that meets your needs. Do not be afraid to ask questions or to get a second opinion.

– Most of all believe you will be healed, pray for healing, ask those around you to pray for you, and do not give up!

Notes

1. "Stress Management," Mayo Clinic, http://www.mayoclinic.org/healthy-living/stress-management/in-depth/positive-thinking/art 200439 50 (accessed March 1, 2015, 1-2).
2. "Prayer and healing: A Medical and Scientific Perspective on Randomized Controlled Trials," by Chittaranjan Andrade and Rajiv Radhakrishnan. Indian Journal of Psychiatry, 2009 Oct-Dec; 51(4): 247253.doi, http://www.ncbi.nlm.nih.gov/pmc/articles/PMC280 2370 (accessed March 1, 2015, 1).

CHAPTER 8

Eating Cancer To Death

My people perish for lack of knowledge.
—Hosea 4:6

Arctic air is howling across the frozen landscape like a starved animal. It is 6:00 am. The Inuk scarcely sees the trail, but his malamutes are cousins of the wolf and have keen vision. Suddenly he brings the sled to a stop, at the exact spot wolves had killed one of his dogs. Jumping off the sled he lays down the wolf bait, a hand full of frozen-blocks of fresh blood. Hidden inside are chips of flint and bone, honed to razor sharp edges. If the wolves take the bait they will lacerate their tongues and spill fresh blood on the block—an invitation to lick more wildly. Swallowing the bait is even more lethal. The Inuk realize it is a cruel method, but the wilderness is unforgiving. Who would not exploit the weakness of the thing that will try to kill again?

Cancer can be even more ominous than a pack of hungry wolves, because its nature is to feed off normal tissue in the body until it chokes the body to death. Worse, it kills indiscriminately. Nevertheless, cancer has abnormal metabolic characteristics, which are not widely known. Cancer has a huge appetite for sugar; it is not able to process fats for metabolism; it's growth is promoted by diets high in animal protein and casein, which is a specific protein only found in cow's milk; and cancer cannot live without methionine, one of the essential amino acids. As the Inuk used fresh blood against the wolf, so we can smartly exploit cancer's metabolic characteristics against it.

This chapter exposes key metabolic characteristics of cancer, namely how it processes sugar, fats, diets high in animal-based protein and a protein found in milk called casein, and the essential amino acid—methionine. It then shows how to combine them into a novel anticancer diet—the Hybrid Cancer Diet. If this diet is combined with periodic or intermittent fasting, and if implemented diligently, it has the potential to place extraordinary stress on cancers' ability to grow, with the possibility of even eating it to death. This diet, along with fasting, affords a new angle of attack against cancer that can be used as a complement to either conventional, integrative, or alternative cancer treatment programs, and will amplify the potential effectives of these treatments. Before discussing the metabolic characteristics of cancer, lets first examine some general facts about cancer.

What Is Cancer? Hippocrates, a famous Greek physician of the 5th century B.C, was the first to record cancer. He described it as a crab because it spreads out from a single point and invades the entire body.[1] In Greek Mythology the goddess Hera sent a giant crab to kill Hercules. Hera named the crab after a constellation, Cancer, the Greek word for crab. In the end however, Hercules perceived the crab had a weak spot on its shell, so he crushed it with his foot and prevailed.[2] As Hercules crushed the crab, so can we crush cancer if we know its weak spots.

So why is cancer so dangerous? According to the National Cancer Institute, cancer is a disease where DNA becomes damaged and normal cells transform into abnormal cells, which grow at an out of control rate and invade nearby tissue. Ultimately, the cancer spreads to other areas of the body via the circulatory and lymphatic systems. Cancer is malignant, meaning it invades the body by overtaking and starving it to death. There are four different types of cancer. All four exhibit the same aberrant cellular characteristics.

The Four Types Of Cancer

1. **Carcinomas** involve the epithelial cells of the skin, and membranes that line or cover organs and gland and comprise 90 percent of all cancers. They include cancers of the esophagus, throat, stomach, lung, breast, prostate, brain, nervous system, skin and all other organs.[3]

Melanoma, which means black tumor, is a subcategory of skin cancer. It forms in the epithelial cells of the skin. It is a more dangerous cancer than skin cancer, because it spreads through the pigment-producing cells of the skin.[4]

2. **Sarcoma** forms in the skeletal system, which consists of bone, cartilage, connective tissue, fat, muscle and blood vessels.

3. **Leukemia** is a cancer that forms in the bone marrow and produces large numbers of abnormal cells that spread into the blood.

4. **Lymphoma**, including multiple myeloma, is cancer that takes over the cells that make up the body's immune system.[5]

Key Traits of Cancer: Cancer grows at a hyper metabolic rate—as much as eight times that of normal cells[6], and even faster in certain carcinomas, such as HER2 over-expressive ones—the cancer I had. Cancer cells do not exhibit apoptosis, which is a sort of programmed cell death, while normal cells do. Cancer cells multiply endlessly. It is a ferocious consumer of glucose, which is essentially sugar that is manufactured by the body primarily from carbohydrates and secondarily from protein, but not fats. Glucose is the body's chief source of energy.

Cancer also consumes excessive amounts of nutrients to support its rapid cell division. Because of this, patients with advanced cancer can experience a condition called cachexia, a wasting away syndrome marked by extreme weight loss, muscle atrophy, fatigue, weakness, and significant loss of appetite. In its final stage, the healthy parts of the body slowly starve to death, while the cancer continues to grow.[7]

A cancerous tumor is able to camouflage its rogue nature so that white blood cells are not able to identify and destroy it. The byproduct of cancer cell division is lactic acid. This byproduct produces lots of hydrogen ions and causes the tumor, surrounding tissue, and eventually the entire body, to become highly acidic. A highly acidic body damages the body's immune system, organs and overall health, and accelerates the growth of cancer.

What Causes Cancer? There are generally four categories of factors that cause cancer:

1. <u>Diet and lifestyle</u> factors, such as obesity, poor diet and nutrition, chronic inflammation, smoking, excessive alcohol, lack of exercise, and certain prescription drugs.

2. <u>Environmental</u> factors include viruses or toxins that enter the body as pesticides, heavy metals, industrial chemicals, and preservatives, and additives in food. It can also be caused by exposure to excessive therapeutic radiation, microwaves, ultraviolet light, and electromagnetic energy. Recent research is showing a strong link between root canals and breast cancer. Long-term bacterial infections in the gums, and metal amalgams used in dentistry, are also suspected of causing cancer.

3. <u>Cultural and genetic</u> factors are based on ethnicity and heredity. Ethnicity speaks to cultural behaviors that may increase the risk of cancer passed down via offspring. Genetic factors speak only to predisposition to certain types of cancer because of DNA.

4. <u>Randomness</u>, or statistical variation in cell mutation. This fourth category recently captured a number of headlines in scientific journals and world news. In a study performed by researchers at Johns Hopkins University, they reported that chance, or bad luck, contrary to prior understanding, is more of a factor in the cause of cancer than anything else. They did not dispute lifestyle, environmental or heredity as causative factors, but identified them as less causative than random cell mutations.[8] Others criticize their findings as oversimplified, and pointed out that chance plays a role even when causative factors are at work. There are also many other variables at work that the researchers failed to account for.[9] For instance, in lung cancer, chance is a factor even when causative factors are at work.[10] In other words, even though they see correlations and potential cause and effect, they are faced with a lot of unknowns. The biology and chemistry of the body are extremely complex, and so are the systems and processes within it, which makes medical science a sort of "best guess" science in numerous scenarios.

METABOLIC CHARACTERISTICS OF CANCER

Metabolic Characteristic 1: Sugar And Cancer

Doctor Otto H. Warburg, a world-renowned biochemist of the 20th Century, held that the metabolic process of cancer cells is entirely different than normal cells. He is the recipient of the 1931 Nobel Prize in Physiology for work in this area. In a revised lecture titled "The Prime Cause and Prevention of Cancer" in Lindau, Germany, at the meeting of the Nobel-Laureates on June 30, 1966, Warburg stated the following:

> Cancer, above all other diseases, has countless secondary causes. But, even for cancer, there is only one prime cause. Summarized in a few words, the prime cause of cancer is the replacement of the respiration of oxygen in normal body cells by fermentation of sugar. All normal body cells meet their energy needs by respiration of oxygen, whereas cancer cells meet their energy needs in great part by fermentation. From the standpoint of the physics and chemistry of life, this difference between normal and cancer cells is so great that one can scarcely picture a greater difference. Oxygen gas, the donor of energy in plants and animals is dethroned in the cancer cells and replaced by an energy yielding reaction of the lowest living forms, namely, a fermentation of glucose. [11] —Otto H. Warburg

Warburg also discovered that cancer cells prefer glucose to oxygen for metabolism even when the cellular environment is rich in oxygen. This cellular anomaly remains puzzling to researchers because the use of oxygen in cell metabolism is much more efficient than the use of glucose. Why would cells prefer a less efficient process? According to an article in the Journal of Cell Biology, "It is now recognized that the Warburg effect represents a prominent metabolic characteristic of malignant cells."[12]

Other research seems to support Warburg's findings. Several studies involved in vitro experiments, meaning in a laboratory, concluded that if cancer cells are starved of glucose they ultimately commit apoptosis (cell suicide). This is something that cancer cells do not normally do, making it one of the chief reasons why this disease is so dangerous. These studies also revealed that high concentrations of glucose in laboratory studies might cause alterations in gene expression that cause the tumor to grow. They know glucose is essential for cancer's metabolism, but they are not sure as to how much of a contributing factor glucose plays in stimulating the growth of cancer.[13] Others disagree, and contend that sugar will not promote cancer growth.[14] The argument against the concept that cancer prefers glucose to oxygen for metabolism seems unreasonable, because they don't offer an answer as to what promotes the growth of cancer, other than to say, there is some unknown variable at work. This contention strikes a little anemic in logic.

Nonetheless, there are a number of other studies that support

Warburg. One of the major risk factors for breast cancer is high glucose in the blood, because it stimulates rapid division of breast cells. How does this work? High glucose stimulates the pancreas to release excessive insulin. Excessive insulin not only stimulates uptake of glucose on insulin receptors of breast cells, it stimulates production of free-estrogen and the uptake of estrogen on estrogen receptors of breast cells. Women get a double whammy of rapid cell division of breast cells, greatly increasing their risk of breast cancer. According to Doctor Christine Horner, a surgeon and expert on natural health, women with high insulin levels have a 283 percent higher risk of breast cancer.[15] If you are a woman who has breast cancer and you are eating lots of sugar and refined carbohydrates, you are literally accelerating the progression of your disease. Remember what we learned in a previous chapter, excessive sugar and refined carbohydrates do enormous harm to our immune system and inhibit the body's natural ability to prevent and contain cancer.

Doctor Warburg also theorized that normal cells mutated into cancer cells in a very low oxygen environment, and that a high oxygen environment might harm them. Many use Warburg's theory to hypothesize that the root cause of cancer is a low oxygen environment. However, the American Cancer Society begs to differ, and claims more recent evidence does not validate claims that cancer can only form in an oxygen-deprived environment, or that an oxygen rich environment can harm cancer.[16] Yet, various alternative cancer treatment centers claim success in using hyberbaric oxygen chambers to slow the progression of cancer and reduce tumor size. They site studies done on animals, which suggest oxygen therapy might be an effective therapy on humans. This area of medical science remains controversial.

Inflammation is a well-known causative factor in cancer due to reduced circulation. Therefore, Warburg's analysis is sound. A low oxygen environment may not be a primary causative agent of cancer, but it might be one of a number of prerequisite conditions for cancer to not only form, but also to thrive under. I tend to lean towards the "more oxygen is better" scientific camp, and devour as much oxygen as I possibly can in the form of daily exercise, because it supports the immune function, and helps the body reduce inflammation, expels toxins, and makes our body less acidic.

Aside from the controversy surrounding oxygen therapy, Warburg's research on the abnormal cell behavior of cancer is credited with the development of the Positron Emission Tomography (PET) scan. The PET scan is one of the most valuable non-surgical diagnostic tests available to locate cancer, to measure the intensity of its metabolic rate, and to more accurately stage the disease.

PET Scan: PET scans are important diagnostic tests used to stage most cancers. They are sometimes combined with a Computed Tomography (CT) scan and are called CT-PET scans. A PET scan uses a small amount of radioactive material to help reveal the location of the tumor. It provides accurate location, size and metabolic intensity information to perform biopsies, surgeries, and assign appropriate treatment protocols. A PET scan is not a perfect diagnostic tool and does not see every cancer cell in the body, but only areas where high metabolic activity is present.

How does it work? In a PET scan, short-lived positron-emitting radioisotopes are mixed with a glucose solution and they bond together into molecules. The radioactive-glucose mixture is then administered intravenously into the blood after the patient fasts for six hours to ensure a low blood-sugar level. The patient is also required to sit still for at least one hour prior to the test to afford the cancer cells less competition with normal cells in absorbing glucose. As the radioisotopes decay, positrons are released that strike electrons and produce gamma rays. The gamma rays radiate in every direction inside out from the tumor and are picked up by radiation sensitive film outside the body. In comparison, the CT scan radiates X-rays outside in to the body to produce images of tissue and organs. The PET and CT scans can be used independently, or they can be overlaid to produce a three dimensional computer image with the locations of any areas that have a high metabolic rate, such as cancer.[17]

PET scans need to be carefully evaluated by both radiologists and oncologists because serious viral and bacterial infections, such as pneumonia, exhibit high metabolic rates and can be misdiagnosed as cancer. This made me wonder if there is actually some merit behind an old adage that says, "feed a cold and starve a fever." Feeding a cold with the right foods bolsters the immune system and fends off the cold. Starving a fever deprives a raging bacterial or viral infection of glucose, lending scientific credence to this old adage.

Since we just learned that cancer loves sugar and has a metabolic rate much greater than normal cells, it seems appropriate to make an effort to deny it the thing it loves most. However, this is only one piece of the metabolic puzzle on how to eat cancer to death. Cancer can still get glucose from proteins in our diet, and also when the body converts muscle tissue to glucose. Further, our liver takes lactic acid produced by both muscle and cancer, converts it to glucose, and then reintroduces it back into the blood stream. So even if we deny our body sugar, carbohydrates and protein, cancer can still find some energy from lactic acid. This process dispels a myth that continues to circulate among some health websites on the Internet. This is not to say that we should not be on a no sugar, low carbohydrate diet when we have cancer. Any effort to bring glucose and insulin levels down helps slow the rate of growth of the tumor and is worthwhile.

Nevertheless, there is much more to the metabolic story of cancer that we will explore next. Are you ready? Lets dive in and explore another fascinating metabolic characteristic of cancer.

Metabolic Characteristic 2: Fats And Cancer

Of the three macronutrients used by normal cells: glucose, lipids (fats) and protein—fats are the only source of energy that cancer is not able to use for energy. One might surmise that a cancer patient who eats nothing but fats for a time could literally eat their cancer to death. Theoretically this is true, but such a diet is not sustainable for an extended period of time because the body needs all three macronutrients to function properly.

The conversion of fats to energy is a chemical process called ketosis. When fats go through ketosis they produce ketones, which normal cells can use for energy—but not cancer cells. Using this metabolic characteristic of cancer as a therapy became known as the Ketogenic diet. The Ketogenic diet was first made popular by Doctor Russell Wilder, at the Mayo Clinic in 1924, for treating epilepsy, especially in children. It was subsequently supplanted by pharmaceuticals. Although, it never completely died and others have continued Doctor Wilder's work using ketosis as a therapy. The Charlie Foundation promotes the Ketogenic diet for treating epilepsy worldwide. Another example is Dominic D'Agostino, PhD., of the University of South Florida. He is a pioneer in studying metabolic therapies for treating neurological disorders, brain cancer, and metastatic cancer. Doctor D'Agostino has produced some fascinating work in the laboratory using the Ketogenic diet, ketone supplements and hyperbaric oxygen therapy as a means to slow the metastatic growth of cancer in mice and prolong life. He also has some interesting videos on YouTube explaining the Ketogenic diet and knows of a number of cancer patients who have gone on this diet with significantly improved outcomes. He is clearly a big proponent of the metabolic theory of cancer as a means of developing safer and more effective treatments. The metabolic theory of cancer however, is not widely accepted in conventional cancer circles.

The Ketogenic diet is also widely used as a weight loss diet by those who do not have cancer. It can bring glucose levels down. It is essentially an alkaline diet that is very high in fat, low in carbohydrates and low in protein.

When used in the context of treating cancer, the Ketogenic diet does not attempt to completely deplete the body of glucose, but to make ketones the prominent energy source. At a minimum, the Ketogenic diet will challenge the ability of cancer to grow, and may even trigger cancer cell suicide, which would reverse its growth. This diet is being promoted my many Naturopathic Doctors, and integrative and alternative cancer centers across the country. In addition to a Ketogenic diet, with Intermittent Fasting, whereby all of one's daily calories are consumed in a four to six hour window during the day; for example, between 10:00 am and 4:00 pm. This approach allows the body to enter into ketosis much faster and works synergistically with any type of cancer therapy, both conventional and alternative.

The problem with this diet however, is that you have to train your body to depend upon ketones, instead of glucose and protein for most of its energy. This can take a lot of time and exceptional eating discipline—and so it is with every other sort of cancer diet. Furthermore, to determine if the body has entered a state of ketosis, one has to take semi-weekly measurements of blood glucose and ketone levels. Naysayers argue that this diet is unhealthy because it is unbalanced, not sustainable and that too much fat in the diet promotes insulin resistance, which is the inability of cells to properly absorb glucose, resulting in excessive blood sugar. If the body doesn't discover how to depend more on fats than glucose for metabolism, then this diet could potentially backfire and promote cancer growth instead.

So what kind of fats should one eat on a Ketogenic diet? This is sort of a slippery question. In general, we should take a well-informed and balanced approach in the consumption of fats. First, cut out all trans fats, which are partially hydrogenated oils, found in margarine and shortenings. Although one can eat trans fats on any sort of cancer diet, they are not heart healthy if eaten on a regular basis. The same can be said for the saturated fats found in animal meats, dairy, eggs, and fish. These foods should be off limits on a cancer diet anyhow, and the reason why will be explained in the next two sections. Saturated fats are also found in coconut oil and palm kernel oil, which are considered by many to have healthier types of saturated fat. For those who claim fish is needed to get adequate amounts of Omega 3, you can always take fish oil or flaxseed oil instead. Olive oil is loaded with heart healthy Omega 9's, so one can eat as much of this as one likes. All of the Omega 6 oils are safe to consume too, as long as they are not consumed at more than a 2:1 ratio with Omega 3's, to avoid the risk of systemic inflammation. In short, all types of fats are fair game, but the animal proteins that go with them are not.

Although some people who have gone on a Ketogenic diet claim they experienced regression of their tumor and even remission of the disease, there are other aspects of the metabolic characteristics of cancer that can be used smartly with the concept behind the Ketogenic diet. Let's discuss these metabolic characteristics next.

Metabolic Characteristic 3: Animal Protein, Casein and Cancer

Doctors T. Colin Campbell and Thomas Campbell performed the largest study ever on the effects of diet and disease and published their results in multiple peer reviewed journals, and in a book titled *The China Study*. The New York Times touted their work as the "Grand Prix of Epidemiology." It is the most far-reaching study ever accomplished that shows a convincing association between multiple diseases and those on a high animal-based protein diet.

Specifically, people who consumed predominantly plant based foods experienced remarkably less chronic disease than those on more animal based diets. They believe animal based proteins are the culprits. Extensive laboratory studies indicate, "Low-protein diets inhibited the initiation of cancer by Aflatoxin, regardless of how much of this carcinogen was administered . . ."[18] **They found that low animal-based protein diets dramatically blocked cancer growth, and that they could turn cancer growth on and off simply by changing the level of animal protein consumed.** All proteins exhibited this effect. However, one protein distinguished itself above all the others, a protein called casein, which comprises 87 percent of cow's milk, in that it promoted all stages of the cancer process. The proteins that did not promote cancer, even at high levels of consumption, were plant-based proteins.[19] This amazing research on animal versus plant-based protein was presented to various government agencies, but under intense lobbying from the food industry their findings were marginalized and ignored.

The principal takeaways are clear. If you know you have cancer, stay away from dairy products and a high animal-based protein diet. The next section validates the results of the China Study even further, particularly in regard to cancer. Now it's time to take a look at methionine, an amino acid found in very high concentrations in the protein of animals, fish, dairy, eggs, seaweed and most nuts. What you see might surprise you.

Metabolic Characteristic 4: Methionine And Cancer

Now that we have examined how sugar, fats, casein, and diets high in animal based protein affect the metabolism of cancer, it's time to take a look at methionine. As you do, please keep in mind one of the major findings of *The China Study*. Researchers could turn cancer growth on and off simply by changing the level of animal protein consumed. Methionine is likely the reason why, even though they did not focus on this amino acid in their research.

Methionine is one of the nine essential amino acids, which are the fundamental building blocks of protein. Please note that there is a debate going on in the protein science community on whether there are eight or nine essential amino acids. This dispute is not important to our discussion on methionine.

The essential amino acids assist in multiple bodily functions, such as manufacturing muscle, repairing wounds, and in transporting nutrients. Methionine is unique in that it is the only amino acid that contains sulfur and it is needed for cell reproduction, specifically protein and RNA synthesis. It is also the requisite substance in the production of several other amino acids, namely homocysteine, cysteine and taurine. What sets it apart even further is that it is the only essential amino acid that can be deprived from diet for prolonged periods of time and is compatible with life.[20] This is because normal cells can remethylate (convert) homocysteine back into methionine for cell reproduction. In contrast, cancer cells do not have the ability to remethylate homocysteine.[21] This has been proven in laboratory studies, which demonstrate methionine-deprived cancer cells will die even when homocysteine is present. Moreover, for over 40 years researchers have tested various cancers in the laboratory with amino acids, using both animal and human cancer cells. All of these studies produced identical results, showing that out of all of the amino acids, methionine was the only one that caused cancer cells to die when deprived of it. It seems methionine, more than any other amino acid, plays an irreplaceable role in not only the growth of cancer cells but also their survivability. Some researchers are even claiming, "Methionine dependence is the only known general metabolic defect in cancer."[22]

A handful of Phase I clinical studies have demonstrated the safety of a methionine restricted diet. These studies were also isocaloric. An isocaloric diet is popular among bodybuilders, because it allows weight loss without muscle loss. It permits one to eat whatever they want as long as they consume the same amount of protein, carbohydrates and fats each day.[23]

Researchers at Baylor College of Medicine in Houston, Texas, reinforced what prior research showed. Cancer cells die when they are denied methionine. In a Phase I clinical trial done in 2002, they examined eight metastatic cancer patients who were on feeding tubes to see whether restricting methionine in their diet was safe and whether it would bring down levels of it in their blood. On both accounts the answer was yes. The diet was isocaloric and consisted of moderate protein that was methionine restricted, moderate carbohydrates and fat, for a total of 2,500 to 3,500 calories per day. They used a commercial protein powder that is methionine free but rich in all the other essential amino acids, called **Hominex-2** Amino Acid Modified Medical Food. They restricted methionine consumption to two mg per kg of patient weight, per day, for an average of 17 weeks. A different way to frame this number is 0.9 mg of methionine per 1 pound of body weight. A simple rule of thumb is to multiply body weight by 0.9 to get a level consistent with the study. This means that a 150-pound person was restricted to 135 mg of methionine per day. On average, patients lost only one pound of weight per week.

In regard to average weight lost, keep in mind that the health of these patients was already severely compromised. After only two weeks on the restricted diet, methionine levels dropped 58 percent.[24]

The researchers in this study also demonstrated that a diet restricted in methionine placed significant stress on cancers' ability to grow. The lead researcher said,

> Numerous in vitro and animal studies demonstrate the effectiveness of dietary methionine restriction in inhibiting growth and eventually causing death of cancer cells. In contrast, normal host tissues are relatively resistant to methionine restriction. . . . In addition, the trial has yielded some preliminary evidence of antitumor activity. One patient with hormone-independent prostate cancer experienced a 25% reduction in serum prostate specific antigen (PSA) after 12 weeks on the diet, and a second patient with renal cell [kidney] cancer experienced an objective radiographic response [the tumor died]. The possibility that methionine restriction may act synergistically with other cancer treatments such as chemotherapy, is being explored.[25]

What is so interesting about the findings of this study is that it was a Phase I clinical trial that focused on the safety of a methionine restricted diet. It was entirely incidental that they discovered 25% reduction in PSA in one prostrate cancer patient after only 12 weeks, and regression of a tumor in a patient with renal cancer to the extent it was not radiographically detectable. Keep in mind that these patients all had advanced stages of cancer. It begs the question of why haven't there been Phase II and III trials that examine the effectiveness of a methionine-restricted diet in a double blind controlled setting. Another point worth noting is that this study concluded that it was safe to restrict methionine in the diet of severely compromised cancer patients for up to 39 weeks. If 0.9 mg of methionine per 1 pound of body weight is safe for up to 39 weeks, and there was evidence of partial and complete regression of tumors in several patients, what might be the impact of restricting methionine by much more over a shorter period of time?

It seems reasonable to ask whether there is a period of time where a certain level of methionine restriction will cause a rapid death of the tumor? I think most other cancer patients would want to know the answer. If we knew that rapid cancer cell death could start occurring in as little as three days of complete methionine restriction, I'd be the first to sign up for a three plus day water fast. It's hard to believe that the researchers in the aforementioned study didn't ponder this same question. What are the research money gods afraid of?

In other research, a synthetic enzyme called methioninase was developed to inhibit methionine use by cells in the body. This research was an effort to determine if a drug could be developed that would provide a safer alternative than restricting a patient's diet. This was based on a presumption within the cancer research and regulating culture that a methionine-restricted diet is a dangerous approach to treating cancer. This would be the argument of the large pharmaceutical companies as well, since they fund huge portions of cancer research. In any case, they discovered that methioninase produced serious side effects and concluded, "Because of potential toxicity and quality of life problems, prolonged methionine restriction with diet or with methioninase is not suitable for clinical use. Methionine restriction may find greater application in association with various chemo-therapeutic agents."[26] Numerous experimental results accumulated during the last three decades suggest that methionine restriction can become an additional therapeutic strategy, notably in association with chemotherapy.[27]

It's interesting that they concluded that a methionine-restricted diet was not safe, when that was not the subject of their study. The biases, false assumptions, generalizations and false conclusions within the research community are at times not difficult to find the more one reads their literature. What's even more distressing is that this report was written in 2003, and there has not yet been an FDA approved treatment that exploits this spectacular weakness of cancer.

That said, methionine is found in high concentrations in the following foods, from the highest to the lowest: seaweed, sesame seeds, meats, dairy, fish, shellfish, eggs, followed by nuts, grains, rice and beans, with the lowest found in vegetables and fruits. Some nuts and beans are deceptively high in methionine, such as Brazil nuts and soybeans, respectively. Green peas, lentils, corn, avocados and pinto beans are fairly low in methionine, all of which are high in other plant-based proteins. For a breakdown of milligrams of methionine per type of food see **Appendix C**.

There are a number of testimonies on the Internet by those who claim they went on a carrot or beet juice diet and it put their cancer into remission. Most would dismiss this as anecdotal and therefore unreliable. But if they understood the validity of the science behind methionine restriction, it might cause them to take a second look. There are numerous testimonies of people that have gone on some sort of vegan or juicing diet, who experienced remarkable results. I believe it's not the nutrients in the vegetarian diet that are causing these excellent outcomes, but it's the fact that a vegan diet is by definition a methionine-restricted diet.

For those who are interested in a more formal approach to implementing a methionine-restricted diet, the Nori Protocol is available, which requires the supervision of a doctor and has a cost associated with it. This protocol greatly restricts methionine for seven to ten days and then allows consumption of foods with low to moderate levels of methionine for three to four days, like almonds and pinto beans. It then cycles back to a highly restricted methionine diet for another seven to ten days. During the off days, dieters consume moderately high doses of sodium selenite, a form of selenium, while they replenish their body with methionine. Dieters are encouraged to eat foods high in natural digestive enzymes, such as tropical fruit, because it is believed they help make cancer cells more susceptible to the sodium selenite. This Protocol can only be done under the supervision of a Doctor and is discussed in more detail in Chapter 14.

THE HYBRID CANCER DIET

Why not take the four metabolic characteristics of cancer that we just learned about and combine them into a Hybrid Cancer Diet? Following is a summary of what this diet looks like.

1. Eliminate sugar and consume a balance of fruits and vegetables. It might seem contradictory to restrict sugar entirely while allowing fruits. To some extent this holds true, but some experts believe it is much more important to bring methionine down than it is to bring sugar down. Certainly, bringing both down at the same time will produce the greatest anticancer effect.

There are some foods that are low in carbohydrates, high in fat and low in methionine, such as olives and macadamia nuts. Almond butter is also low in carbohydrates, high in fat, high in amino acids, but still relatively low in methionine. A high fruit diet is not advisable for someone that is insulin resistant or diabetic. There exist a number of fruits with much less fructose content then others, which will help keep total glucose consumption lower. See **Appendix D** for a table showing a list of popular Fruits By Level Of Sugar.

2. No animal or fish based protein. Only eat small portions of plant-based protein that is low in methionine.

3. No Dairy. Dairy is loaded with both casein and methionine.

4. Moderate to high level of plant based oils. The Ketogenic diet strives for 50 to 60 percent of daily caloric intake to be from good oils. Training the body to use more oil for metabolism takes time. Anyone who starts this diet can easily shoot for something less aggressive, like 30 to 40 percent of diet. Recall, a diet too high in fat and carbs might promote insulin resistance, and if protein isn't restricted sufficiently it could actually backfire and stimulate the growth of the tumor.

5. Other Protein: I've used an organic protein powder to supplement my diet for almost two years, called Vegan Smart. One scoop has 10 grams of all the essential amino acids, probiotics, digestive enzymes and lots of other vitamins and nutrients in it, and only 109 mg of methionine. However, if you have the budget, HOMINEX-2 is a much better option than Vegan Smart, since it is a methionine free protein powder. Remember, this product was proven to be safe and effective in the Baylor College study.

Although HOMINEX-2 is pricey, it's an excellent supplement for any sort of anticancer diet. It's sold on Amazon and EBay, but is less expensive at **VitalityMedical.com.** The best option from a price point of view is to purchase HOMINEX-2 at the manufacture's website, **Abbottnutrition.com**, because it is much cheaper than the other three stores. The only catch is that Abbott's website requires the customer to check a block that claims they have a prescription from a doctor for their product prior to making a purchase.

Therapeutic Level Of Methionine

The therapeutic level for an extended low methionine diet is referenced in the previously discussed clinical study of metastatic cancer patients done by Baylor College. The level they tested was no more than 0.9 mg of methionine for every pound of patient weight. For example, a patient that weighs 100 pounds would restrict their diet to 90 mg of methionine per day. So how much methionine does the body require per day? One study indicates that the amount of methionine a body needs to remain healthy is approximately 6.5 mg per pound of weight, per day. For a person weighing 150 pounds this would equal 975 mg per day.[28]

Theoretically, one could eat salads and vegetables with healthy oils, low sugar content fruits, plant based protein powder, and various vegetable and fruit juices for long periods of time with no weight loss.

One could also go on a water only fast for one or two days at a time to drive the methionine level in the blood down quickly.

A diet that is restricted in sugar, carbohydrates, casein, and methionine, will provide an opportunity to place significant stress on cancers' ability to grow and potentially down stage a tumor, which would make it easier to treat and improve the prognosis.

Although the Hybrid Cancer Diet can be used as a stand-alone therapy, it can also be a powerful complement to a conventional, integrative or alternative cancer treatment program. Using nutrition to treat cancer is highly dependent upon a very disciplined approach to eating, something that can be learned if practiced.

Fasting And Cancer

Those wishing to have an immediate impact on their cancer using nutritional therapy that exploits the metabolic abnormalities of cancer should consider doing a water-only or calorie restricted fast. Regular fasting has all sorts of benefits, such as detoxifying the colon and other organs, reducing inflammation, insulin resistance and diabetes, and autoimmune disease symptoms. It can also help the body repair damaged tissue. One study showed that depriving the body of methionine for a 24-hour period reduced the circulating methionine in the blood by an average of 58 percent.[29] This is corroborated by research done in the laboratory that showed if cancer cells are completely deprived of methionine for 24 hours in a petri dish, they die off dramatically. It seems that complete deprivation of methionine will produce an intense die off of cancer cells to the point that it could kill the tumor. How many days of fasting this might require is anyone's guess. One can surmise that the longer one fasts the more likely one is likely to instigate a massive die off of cancer cells. If a tumor dies too quickly however, it can create a dangerous condition called Tumor Lysis Syndrome (TLS). In TLS, tumor cells release high levels of potassium phosphate and nucleic acid into the body and can cause all kinds of serious conditions, such as metabolic acidosis, kidney injury and heart failure. So serious attempts at water only fasts for extended periods of time should only be done under the supervision of a doctor.

When I first discovered I had cancer I went on a two-day water fast followed by a calorie restricted vegan diet, which I believe was instrumental in reversing the growth of my tumor. For cancer patients who are severely compromised from conventional treatment, a calorie-restricted diet is not feasible. Maintaining some level of daily exercise is also beneficial during periods of fasting. Among other things, exercise oxygenates the body, bolsters the immune system, purges toxins, and improves emotional and mental quality of life—and equally so, it places a much greater burden on the amount of methionine and glucose available to the cancer. Psychologically, exercise gives us a competitive edge against our disease. I gained a sense of empowerment knowing that the sweat on my brow from exercising put stress on cancer's ability to grow. I wanted to starve it to death. Even the thought of making it suffer, however fanciful it might sound, produced a sense of satisfaction. To my surprise, I was able to go on and off a seven-day calorie restricted and low methionine diet without losing more than a couple of pounds. By calorie restricted I mean 800-1000 calories a day.

Another form of a calorie-restricted diet is Intermittent Fasting, which places the body into a fasting state every day. It will place the body into a state of ketosis much faster than a calorie restricted diet. It requires one to keep all eating within a four or so hour window, let's say from 12:00 to 4:00 pm. If it's too difficult to maintain, then modify it to five or six hours. Intermittent Fasting also necessitates one to drink lots of water during the non-eating hours. When I tried doing this I found myself cheating a little bit by eating a small snack or two during the non-eating hours. I figured, if you have to cheat a little, then so be it, since it's vastly better than doing nothing. We don't have to perform these anticancer eating protocols perfectly; we just have to place ourselves in a better position than we were before.

Another option is to cycle between a calorie-restricted diet and intermittent fasting every second or third day, or even just once a week.

This is the approach that worked best for me, because I was more focused on restricting milligrams of methionine than calories.

I have encountered numerous cancer patients with amazing testimonies on how they managed the growth of their cancer using nutritional therapy and fasting—and some like myself would add daily exercise. In one case, a cousin of mine, Ms. L., with Stage 2 breast cancer, went on a semi-Ketogenic, low methionine diet, patterned after what I did. She was on this diet for three-months, while waiting to get insurance, diagnostics and a treatment plan in place. Pathology characterized here cancer as a HER 2 triple overexpressed adenocarcinoma, which is one of the most aggressive types of cancer. Her doctor told her that she would need surgery, followed by either radiation or chemo. To her doctor's surprise, her tumor did not grow at all during the three-months she waited for surgery. They removed the tumor and found no sign of other cancer in her body, and decided she was no longer a candidate for radiation or chemo.

In another instance, Ms. R., who had Stage 3 breast cancer, did not have insurance and was trying to manage her cancer with a vegan diet, high dose intravenous Vitamin C, and natural substance therapy. I met her at an integrative cancer center that I was attending also. I explained to her the power of a low methionine diet and fasting, so she modified her diet further and made it through a six-day water-only fast. She was in excellent condition and had not been compromised by conventional cancer therapy when she went on this fast. She also took daily walks during the fast. Within days of completing the fast her breast swelled up and became very tender. She had a fairly large tumor that had already erupted through the skin on the left side of her left breast. The oncologist at this clinic, who had worked in private practice and also for the Cancer Treatment Centers of America for a number of years, physically examined her and diagnosed tumor necrosis. The doctor told Ms. R. that she might experience some drainage from the tumor. The tumor subsequently released over 30 ounces of fluid.

Another person I know, Mr. H., who was on a low methionine juicing diet for over a year experienced the disappearance of numerous metastatic lesions on his liver. During this period he was also boosted his immune system with natural substances and received high dose intravenous Vitamin C. Although all of these testimonies are anecdotal, there remains a strong correlation to what they did with diet, exercise, natural substances and fasting, and an improved prognosis.

Traditional Oncology Versus Cancer Diets

Using the metabolic characteristics of cancer as a complementary element of a broader cancer treatment program is gaining wider acceptance in traditional oncology. For example, in 2012, Craig P. Thompson, President and CEO of Memorial Sloan Kettering made the following statement in a presentation he gave on, "How Do People Get Cancer". He said, "If you overfeed someone with fat, you don't increase their cancer risk at all. If you overfeed someone with carbohydrates, you dramatically increase their cancer risk. Protein is half way in between."[30]

Even though Mr. Thompson is speaking about the causes of cancer and preventing it, he is clear in stating that a high fat diet may reduce the risk of getting cancer. It indirectly gives some validation to the science that says cancer cells are not able to use ketones from fats for cell metabolism. At any rate, many traditional practitioners continue to shun any sort of cancer diet.

Advocates of cancer diets criticize traditional medicine for spending decades of time and enormous amounts of public and private funding on the genome project, falsely identifying cancer as a genetic disease. They claim traditional cancer research will never find a cure through genetic research, because cancer is a metabolic disease not a genetic one, except in a few rare forms of cancer.

Supporters of treating cancer with diet argue it is not only safe, but also extremely effective in inhibiting the growth of cancer. These testimonies reinforce the findings of numerous studies done in the laboratory. With that said, it still involves a major dietary change, which may be problematic for many. This is why every cancer patient should be consulting with a Nutritionist.

Over the last two years, I brought my findings on the scientific research surrounding cancer cell death through methionine deprivation to a handful of Naturopathic doctors and nurses, two integrative oncologists, and an anti-aging doctor, all of whom were treating cancer patients, including myself at some point—and surprisingly, not a single one of them were aware of the clinical studies and the laboratory experiments that indicate methionine deprivation can kill cancer cells. All of them, except for the anti-aging doctor, were promoting a

Ketogenic diet as the state of the art in alternative anticancer nutritional therapy. I also found this to be true with other integrative and alternative cancer centers that I consulted with. Be that as it may, a vegetarian, low methionine, moderately high in fat diet is the foundation of my personal treatment plan.

Call this anecdotal if you wish, but the only late-stage metastatic cancer patients that I have encountered over the last four years, who have survived well beyond the statistics, are ones that were on some sort of vegetarian or juicing diet—not a ketogenic one.

Summary

We learned some remarkable things in this chapter about cancer's weaknesses; namely, its voracious appetite for sugar, its inability to use fats for cell metabolism, how casein and high animal based protein diets promote its growth, and its critical need for methionine. This information can be wisely used against cancer, just like the Inuk used the wolves' lust for blood against it. Diet can now be viewed as something much more valuable to us than just sustenance. It can be used as a formidable weapon to attack cancer from a different angle, and it can provide a safe and effective complement to any cancer treatment program.

I tried to starve my cancer in a smart way, while maintaining a healthy diet, because I declared war on it. What I did with my cancer diet was entirely safe for me and I felt extraordinarily empowered each day, knowing that I was fighting back. Unfortunately, I knew very little about the metabolic characteristics of cancer until much later. To my good fortune, however, the vegan cancer diet I implemented prior to entering treatment was very similar to the Hybrid Cancer Diet. I believe this diet, along with fasting, played a huge role in shrinking my tumor by over 250 percent prior to starting treatment. Fasting is also a powerful in nutritional therapy. Research shows that any sort of fasting will stress cancer to some extent every day. Fasting affords an indispensable weapon against cancer and it should be a fundamental component in every personal treatment plan.

For many, treating cancer with food is probably too radical and simplistic an idea to accept at first blush. Or perhaps, the eating discipline required for this diet is beyond one's ability. If so, then at least try to cut out all sugar and reduce intake of white starchy foods.

Also, cut out as much meat, fish and dairy as possible. Any measure one takes to become a more disciplined eater in a manner that puts stress on the cancer's rate of growth is worth the effort. There is absolutely no reason why some sort of cancer diet should not be part of every cancer patient's personal treatment plan. Let's get busy today and start eating cancer to death, one small bite at a time!

Notes

1. Pecorino, Laureen. Why Millions Survive Cancer: The Successes of Science. New York: Oxford University Press, 2011, 73.
2. "Cancer: Windows to the Universe." http://www.windows2universe.org/mythology/cancer.html (accessed February 1, 2015).
3. National Cancer Institute, "Dictionary on Cancer Terms", http://www.cancer.gov/dictionary (accessed January 27, 2015).
4. Ruzic, Neil. Racing to a Cure: A Cancer Victim Refuses Chemotherapy and Finds Tomorrow's Cures In Today's Scientific Laboratories. Urbana and Chicago: University of Illinois Press, 2003, 83.
5. Ibid., NCI, Dictionary on Cancer Terms.
6. Biology Online, Dictionary, http://www.biology-online.org/dictionary/Apoptosis (accessed February 3 2015).
7. Dr. Kevin Connors, "Starving Your Cancer". http://hosted-p0.vresp.com/829231/572a4caa1c/ARCHIVE (accessed January 27, 2015).
8. Bloomberg, "Cancer is More Bad Luck Than Bad Behavior, Study Says", January 2, 2015. http://www.bloomberg.com/news/print2015-0102/cancer-largely-due-to-biolgical-bad-luck-rather-than-behavior.html (accessed January 2, 2015).
9. Science 2 January 2015: Vol. 347 no. 6217 pp. 78-81 DOI:10.1126/science. 1260825, "Variation in cancer risk among tissues can be explained by the number of stem cell divisions",
http://www.sciencemag.org/content/347/6217/78
(accessed February 1, 2015).
10. "On Randomness, Determinism, False Dichotomies and Cancer", Tuesday, January 6, 2015 19:29, http://beforeitsnews.com/science-and-technology/2015/01/on-randomness-determinism-false-dichotomies-and-cancer-2740942.html (accessed February 1, 2015).
11. Revised Lecture titled "The Prime Cause and Prevention of Cancer", Lindau, Germany, at the meeting of the Nobel-Laureates on June 30, 1966, by Otto Warburg, Director, Max Planck-Institute for Cell Physiology, Berlin-Dahlem.
http://healingtools.tripod.com/primecause1.html
(accessed January 27, 2015).
12. "Mitochondrial Respiration Defects in Cancer Cells Cause Activation of Akt Survival Pathway through a Redox-Mediated Mechanism," J Cell Biol. Dec 18, 2006; 175(6): 913–923.
13. "Mythbusters: Complementary and Alternative Treatments in Cancer," Victoria Stern, MA, September 02, 2014, 5.
http://www.medscape.con/viewarticle/830552
(accessed September 14, 2014).

14. Ibid., 6.

15. "High Insulin and Sugar Increases Breast Cancer Risk" by Christine Horner, MD, New Living Magazine. http://www.newliving.com/issues/aug-2005/articles/breast%20cancer.html (accessed June 12, 2015, 1).

16. "Oxygen Therapy", The American Cancer Society, http://www.cancer.org/treatment/treatsmentsandsideeffects/complementaryand alternative medicine/harmacologicalandbiologicaltreatment/oxygen-therapy (accessed February 2, 2015).

17. American Society of Clinical Oncology. "Navigating Cancer Care, Integrated PET-CT Scan", http://www.cancer.net/navigating-cancer-care/diagnosing-cancer/tests-and-procedures/integrated-pet-ct-scan (accessed February 2, 2015).

18. Campbell, Colin T., MD, Campbell, Thomas M., MD. "The China Study." Dallas, Texas: Benbella Books, 2004, 6-7.

19. Ibid.

20. Kaczor, Tina, ND, FABNO, "The Role of Methionine in Cancer Growth and Control," Natural Medicine Journal, Dec 2015 Vol. 7, Issue 12. www.naturalmedicinejournal.com/journal/2015-12/role-methionine-cancer-growth-and-control (accessed January 15, 2018), 1.

21. Ibid.

22. Pavillard V, Drbal AA, Swaine DJ, Phillips RM, Double JA, Nicolaou A. Biochem Pharmacol. Analysis of cell-cycle kinetics and sulfur amino acid metabolism in methionine-dependent tumor cell lines; the effect of homocysteine supplementation. Biochem Pharmacol. 2004;67(8):1587-1599.

23. Hoffman, R.M., "Development of Recombinant Methioninase to Target the General Cancer-Specific Metabolic Defect of Methionine Dependence: a 40-year odyssey," Expert Opin Biol Ther. 2015 Jan;15(1):21-31. Epb 2014 Dec 2, (accessed July 7, 2016).

24. Kaczor, 2.

25. Epner, D.E., et al., Department of Medicine, Baylor College of Medicine "Nutritional Intake and Nutritional Indexes in Adults with Metastatic Cancer on a Phase I Clinical Trial of Dietary Methionine Restriction." NutrCancer. 2002;42(2):158:66. http://www.ncbi.nlm.nih.gov/pubmed/12416254 (accessed July 7, 2016)

26. Epner, D.E., Baylor Department of Medicine, Houston, Texas, "Can Dietary Methionine Restriction Increase the Effectiveness in Chemotherapy in Treatment of Advanced Cancer Patients?", J Am Coll Nutr.2001 Oct:20(5Suppl):443S-449S; discussion 473S-475S. http://www.ncbi.nlm.nih.gov/pubmed/11603655 (accessed July 7, 2016)

27. Cellarier, E. et al., "Methionine Dependency and Cancer Treatment", Cancer Treat Rev. 2003 Dec:29(6):489-99. http://www.ncbi.nim.nih.gov/pubmed/14585259 (accessed July 7, 2016)

28. Ibid.
29. Kaczor, 3.
30. "Why We All Don't Get Cancer", Memorial Sloan-Kettering Cancer Center Posted on Monday, December 17th, 2012 at 3:07 am, by Michael O'Neill. http://ketopia.com/why-we-all-dont-get-cancer-memorial-sloan -kettering-cancer-center (accessed June 11, 2015).

CHAPTER 9

Treatment

I have called upon you every day, O Lord;
I have spread out my hands to you.
—Psalm 89:9

With dread on their faces, a rush of people plodded past each other in a military like cadence through sliding-glass doors, some in steel-clad wheel chairs, while others marched in single file—as if condemned to the gallows. Entering this building is a serious matter and their expressions said so. It was 1:00 pm on November 27, 2013 when we shuffled out of MD Anderson in downtown Orlando. We had been there for over five hours for pre-treatment screening. I am sure I wore a similar woeful countenance earlier that morning as we entered the building.

As Kelly and I silently moved towards the parking garage I remember thinking, "This might be my last stop in life. Would I end up like so many others with cancer and enter into a perpetual cycle of treatments that prolonged my life for a short period of time, yet tethered me to this building until I died? Would I even still be alive a year or two down the road?" I didn't know. But something sweet came upon me that morning. I realized that I was at peace with it all. I had experienced the same peace shortly after I had first been diagnosed with cancer. Somehow it had slipped away in all the hectic activity leading up to the treatment center. How could I not be at peace? I sensed God's love in my heart deeper than ever before. The thought of dying had no power over me that day, nor would it in the challenging days ahead. I was no longer afraid.

The in-processing and pre-treatment evaluation went extremely well.

Now it was time to join our daughter McLain and her family in Charleston, South Carolina for Thanksgiving. We were hoping our other children would be present too, Ryan, Joey and Amy. The five-hour drive would afford us plenty of time to compare notes and contemplate the morning's events.

As we zipped up I-95 I asked Kelly for her observations. She said, "I am really impressed with the doctors and nurses, and I think it is a really good fit for us. I also liked the fact they encouraged us to live on campus during treatment and pointed out that those who try to work during treatment do not fare as well as those who do not." I responded, "I agree. I was also surprised to learn that their program includes consultation with a nutritionist, and family counseling too, if needed. This will give me a chance to compare what I am doing with what they recommend."

We went on to discuss many other things, but one of the biggest issues on both our hearts was how to avoid the surgery. The surgery cannot only kill you, but there are frequently life-long complications to deal with, which significantly impact quality of life. Many who have this surgery are unable to eat normally for the rest of their lives. At that time, we both agreed that it would be better to wait and see the results of the chemo and radiation portion of the program before agreeing to the surgery. In any case, we met with the Oncologist right after the Thanksgiving break.

Chemotherapy

Before we met with the Oncologist, Nurse L. greeted us in the examination room and had us sit down and gave us a seminar on everything you would ever want to know about esophageal cancer. She answered numerous questions about such things as the treatment regimen, the staging of tumors, the types of diagnostic and blood tests I should expect, the side effects of chemo and radiation, and the surgery. She also encouraged us to get a second opinion if we had any reservations about their treatment protocol or if we were uncomfortable in any other way.

The Oncologist would later explain that the treatment consists of a multi-modality regimen, meaning there would be three components to attack the cancer from different directions. It consisted of simultaneous chemo and radiation therapy over a five and one half week period, followed by the surgery, called an esophagectomy. I would receive once a week intravenous (IV) infusions of Carboplatin and Taxol, the chemotherapeutic drugs.

> **Did You Know?**
>
> FDA guidelines stipulate that for a chemotherapy drug to be declared effective it must be able to reduce the size of a tumor by 50 percent over a one-month period. There are no guidelines or mandates that the chemo drug should cure the cancer, it is only used to beat back the cancer.[1] On the other hand, when chemo is combined with radiation therapy it is much more effective than doing the treatments separately.
>
> Surgeons will tell you that chemotherapy alone does not cure cancer, except in some rare instances, where it has proven to put certain cancers into remission, meaning no evidence of the cancer for five years post treatment. These cancers include childhood leukemia, with about an 80 percent success rate for long-term remission, testicular cancer, cutaneous T-cell lymphoma and Hodgkin's disease.[2] Unfortunately, what is left out of many of the positive reports I read on the success of chemotherapy with childhood cancers, is that many children grow up with severe side effects and many others will eventually succumb to a secondary cancer later in life. This is not good enough for me. Why haven't we figured out a way to heal these kids without harming them?

Nurse L. highlighted the need to keep a positive attitude throughout treatment. She also underlined the importance of proper nutrition and daily exercise, even if it meant just taking a walk. Everything she emphasized included things I was already doing, so this really encouraged us. Later, we would get an in depth briefing by Nurse S., who described the chemo drugs I would get, and also some precursor drugs, to help reduce nausea and allergic reactions. During my first chemo session I asked the nurse for the names of all the drugs they were pumping into me, other than the Carboplatin and Taxol.

The precursors included acid reflux and anti-nausea drugs, as well as a steroid and an antihistamine. The precursor drugs are used to trick the body into accepting the toxic chemo agents and inhibit an allergic reaction. I recall thinking, "Are you kidding me! They use precursor drugs to trick the body into accepting the chemo." Even though they have somewhat perfected the cocktail of precursor drugs, there is still a certain percentage of patients that will experience some form of allergic reaction, things ranging from nausea and hives, to anaphylactic shock. Few might know this, but they also deliver a five percent solution of

Dextrose, which is glucose, with the precursor drugs, to stimulate the tumor to gobble up as much chemo as possible—as one might surmise. I stumbled across this fact by reading the labels on my IV bags. It's good to pay attention to everything that is going on with your treatment while in the hospital. The Journal of Patient Safety estimated in 2014 that 210,00 to 440,00 patients suffer a preventable harm that leads to their death as a result of their hospital visit. Followed by heart disease and cancer, mistakes made by hospitals kill more people than anything else in the United States.[3]

After being briefed by both oncology nurses, I met with the Oncologist, Doctor O. He spoke with us for over an hour and was tremendously detailed in answering all of our questions. All of our caretakers at MD Anderson were wonderful. Doctor O. seemed to be particularly interested in my exercise regimen and asked me a number of questions. I told him how often and vigorous I exercise. He said, "Next to a positive attitude and nutrition, exercise is the most important factor in tolerating the treatment and in helping your body resist the cancer and prevent recurrence."

Pathology staged my cancer as a T2bN1Mx tumor, meaning that the stage is a two, the tumor invades the muscularis propria (T2), which is the esophageal muscle, with possibly one lymph node involved (N1), and distant metastasis cannot be assessed (Mx). Please see **Appendix B** for more on staging.

Doctor P., the Gastroenterologist who had performed an ultrasonic endoscopy to stage the tumor said, "This cancer is very challenging because it is like dropping a glass on the floor; tiny shards of glass scatter in every direction and are almost impossible to find." This helped explain why the treatment for esophageal cancer is so aggressive.

Moreover, even if you have a complete response from the treatment, meaning there is no evidence of cancer, studies of breast cancer patients have shown that cancer cells are still circulating in the blood of 50 percent of patients five years following treatment.[4]

I asked Doctor O. about a number of concerns I had about the surgery. He said, "Joe don't worry too much about those things right now. You are scheduled to see the surgeon in a few days, and he is one of the best in this field. He will take you through the paces on what to expect."

I enthusiastically explained to Doctor O. that my acid reflux was cured and that the ultrasonic endoscopy indicated the tumor had shrunk from about 4 cm (1.6 inches) to about 1.5 cm (0.6 inches), and that the Barrett's Esophagus had resolved itself. I said, "You can look at all of my records and see for yourself." I think he found these claims a little too difficult to believe, but I don't blame him. I would later share the regression of my tumor and the healing of Barrett's with the Radiation Oncologist and Surgeon, and their responses were much the same as Doctor O.'s. As far as they were concerned it really did not matter, because the damage to the esophagus caused by the radiation is so severe that the esophagus needs to come out. Ultimately, my doctors insisted that the standard of care required the esophagus to be removed, so it was a moot point. It wasn't moot to me however.

Nevertheless, Doctor O. ended our meeting on a very positive note. He said, "You have a great attitude, you are doing all the right things, and I expect a good outcome for you Joe." In other words, the patient has a very important role to play in how successful the outcome might be, and their effort can make the doctor and nurses jobs a lot easier.

Radiation Therapy

The radiation therapy protocol requires 28 doses of radiation to be spread out over five and one half weeks. The radiation would be delivered daily, Monday through Friday. The absorbed dose would be 50.4 Gy, which is 5,040 rem of radiation. I discovered later that this dosage is 1,000 times greater than the maximum annual safe exposure limit for those who work in a nuclear related occupation, 5,000 mrem. After learning this, I could have used a cardiac massage! Another distressing aspect is that this treatment protocol is a cookie cutter approach, even with the chemotherapy. Everyone gets the maximum dose for their weight, period. Everyone in the cancer industry knows how damaging the treatment is to the human body, but unfortunately, those who treat us have no say over it.

Doctor R., my Radiation Oncologist, explained why they do radiation therapy concurrently with chemo. He stated, "Radiation therapy is overlapped with chemotherapy because the chemo sensitizes the tumor and lymph nodes, making them more susceptible to the radiation." However, the esophagus is one of the most precariously placed parts of the body for radiation therapy, because the liver, kidney, pancreas gall bladder, lungs and heart surround it. In regard to the side

127

effects Doctor R. was very clear. He said,

> The first week or two patients do not experience any serious side
> effects, maybe a little redness on your torso, some nausea and
> fatigue. By week three, most people start noticing red marks on
> their torso, and may have difficulty swallowing food. By week
> four, patients have difficulty swallowing and are on a liquid diet.
> They also start experiencing rashes, and the nausea and fatigue
> are much more pronounced.

I asked, "Is Aloe Vera gel helpful in healing radiation burns?" He said,
"Yes, some people find relief with it, so use whatever works for you." I
read about swallowing pure Aloe Vera gel to help the esophagus heal
but discovered it burned too much and did not use it. Instead, I found
great relief in taking small doses of sodium bicarbonate (Baking Soda)
mixed in water, two to three times daily. In fact, I believe it was the
major factor in allowing me to go the entire five weeks without having
to go on a liquid diet, something Doctor R. and my nurses were
surprised to see. Doctor R. went on to disclose the worst-case
scenarios. He said, "You could lose up to one third of the function of
your liver. You might also lose the function of one kidney. Scar tissue
and inflammation might form in the lower lobes of your lungs."

This was a very intimidating report because I understood that
ionizing radiation damages DNA and can later evolve into radiation-
induced cancer. I also understood the danger of the chemo drugs in
damaging the DNA of cells, not only in my bone marrow, but also in
other areas of my body. At this point, what other choice did I have?

After having read that recurrence of breast and esophageal cancers
typically occurs in the lungs, I asked, "What is the risk of radiation
induced lung cancer?" He said, "There is always a risk of this anytime
we radiate the lung area, but it is not a very high risk, and there is no
way to predict if it will happen." I kind of had an ill feeling in my
stomach when he said this because it validated the risk of radiation
induced lung cancer. I then asked him about the heart, because my
tumor was in an area that places the esophagus right next to the heart.
He said, "There is always a possibility that the heart is exposed to some
radiation." I also asked Doctor R. about other radiation technologies.
One of these treatments is called Brachytherapy, where a small
radioactive substance is inserted into a catheter and endoscopicly placed

near the tumor for a short period. This procedure significantly reduces the amount of collateral damage done to normal tissue, however it does not radiate the lymph nodes and stomach, so it was not an option.

Another treatment, called Proton Therapy, is the latest in radiation technology. It uses protons instead of X-rays to attack the tumor. Most of the radiation is absorbed by the tumor with significantly less collateral damage to normal tissue. The result is a higher tumor kill-rate and a substantial reduction in the risk of damaging local organs and tissue, and in radiation induced cancer. According to the National Cancer Institute, less than one percent of cancer patients in the United States have access to this advanced technology, even though it has been around for over 10 years. The truth behind why there are such long lags in deploying safer and more effective technologies is a profit driven one. Cancer centers need to squeeze every last dollar out of their investments in older technology before they invest in the new.

Surgery

Surgery is considered the most important element in treating tumor related cancers. The Esophagectomy is an extremely radical surgery with life threatening complications. It removes one half to two thirds of the esophagus, and one third to one half of the stomach. The remaining section of the stomach is reconstructed into a tube and pulled up through the solar plexus, which is underneath the lungs, and then reattached behind either the lungs or in the lower neck.

They can also remove 40 lymph nodes or more. Some surgeons believe that the higher the number of lymph nodes removed the higher the survival rate.[5] However, other studies cast some doubt over this belief. Following the surgery, all of the removed parts and lymph nodes are tested for cancer. The post surgery pathology is used to provide a more accurate staging of the cancer, establish a clearer prognosis, and evaluate the effectiveness of the cancer center's treatment protocol.

Nutritional Counseling

As part of MD Anderson's program I received consultation with one of their Nutritionists, Ms. N. One of the most valuable things she did was to validate the supplements I was taking to fight cancer, and help reduce the side effects of chemo-radiation. She also introduced me to vitamin D3 and showed the clinical evidence that proved its ability to significantly reduce the risk of cancer. When I told her I had put myself on curcumin immediately after being diagnosed with cancer, she was surprised. She said, "You are the first patient I have encountered that understands the value of curcumin." She was also surprised that I knew about cancer's appetite for glucose and the science behind the PET scan, and encouraged me to continue my avoidance of sugar.

Ms. N. reinforced the value of daily exercise, but like my nurses, she was concerned that I might experience muscle wasting and recommended I take HMB as a supplement, which is used by weight lifters to build and retain muscle mass.

Additional Medical Counseling

In addition to a nutritionist I decided to see my chiropractor, Doctor T. in Charleston, South Carolina. I was able to see him right before I started treatment. Even though he was not a part of the cancer treatment center's program, I made him a key part of my initial personal treatment plan. Although Doctor T. does not specifically treat cancer patients, he treats the whole body and made some great recommendations on how to detoxify the colon and body before starting treatment. He identified some mineral deficiencies in my diet, and he reinforced my plan to continue an alkaline diet, daily exercise, and the natural supplements I was taking. In particular, he encouraged me to research pancreatic enzymes and how the late Doctor Gonzalez and other naturopathic doctors are using them to fight cancer. Many of Doctor Gonzalez's late-stage pancreatic patients have amazing testimonies in regard to being healed with high dose pancreatic enzymes. After I visited Doctor T., I felt as if I had done everything I possibly could to prepare myself for treatment and to provide my body with the best possible support to heal. I paid out of pocket for his services but it was worth every penny.

Summary

Being processed into a cancer treatment center is a monumental event. I had a hyper-metabolic cancer that came with an ugly five-year survival statistic. I was afraid of the tri-modality treatment and the harm it would inflict on my body. The pressure to do the surgery as the third prong of the standard of care was enormous; yet I hoped and prayed for a way out of it.

As bad as the situation looked, there were some incredible things at work—things that afforded me hope. First, the tumor had not grown during the month preceding treatment; instead, it regressed. Second, the Barrett's Esophagus had resolved itself between the November 12th and December 4th endoscopies, something unheard of. I believe the alkaline diet and the daily use of baking soda to soak the esophagus, helped to cure the Barrett's. How could I not help but believe that prayer, a positive expectation to be healed, and the complementary components of my personal treatment plan all played an important role. My peace had returned to me the morning of November 27th. I felt the Lord's presence. I lifted up my hands. He was near to me—no matter what happened. What greater thing can we experience each day, in this life, than to be at peace.

Notes

1. Ruzic, Neil. "Racing to a Cure: A Cancer Victim Refuses Chemotherapy and Finds Tomorrow's Cures inn Today's Scientific Laboratories." University of Illinois Press: Urbana and Chicago, copyright 2000, 31-32.
2. Ibid.
3. Allen, Marshall, "How Many Die From Medical Mistakes Made In Hospitals,", Scientific American, ProPublica September 20, 2013 https://www.scientificamerican.com/article/how-many-die-from -medical-mistakes-in-us-hospitals/
(accessed November 20, 2016).
4. Somers, Suzanne. Forwarded by Julian Whitaker, MD. "Knockout: Inter -views with Doctors Who Are Curing Cancer – And How to Prevent Get -ting It In The First Place. Crown Publishers: New York, 2009, 158.
5. "Is the Number of Lymph Nodes Removed and the Type of Resection Associated with Postoperative Complications after Esophagectomy for Esophageal Cancer? Arzu Oezcelik et. al., Abstract TU1637. https://www.deepdyve.com/lp/elsevier/is-the-number-of-lymph-nodes-removed-and-the-type-of-resection-V0T0Yk0cih
(accessed November 17, 2015).

CHAPTER 10

Exercise And Cancer

The harder you work, the harder it is to surrender.
—Vince Lombardi

O ncologists and nurses are reluctant to talk too much about survival statistics. I asked my Oncologist what my chance of survival was during our first meeting and he did not give me one. Instead, he said, "It's difficult to tell because you may have lymph node involvement, which would change things; but since you are fit, eat well, have a positive attitude, and exercise regularly you should do better than most." He went on to underscore the value of exercise in helping patients tolerate treatment. This validated the things I did on my own after being diagnosed with cancer. Nonetheless, he remained reluctant to talk about statistics, and for good reason.

Predicting outcomes of patients who undergo simultaneous chemo and radiation therapy, followed by a radical surgery is like trying to nail a bowl of Jell-O to the wall. Doctors and nurses never know for sure whether any particular patient will end up in the statistic that is really good, or the statistic that is not so good. Some patients don't complete chemo-radiation because they become too ill. Others complete chemo-radiation but suffer a complication that excludes them from surgery. Yet, others make it through surgery but succumb to a secondary cancer down the road. No matter how you dice the Jell-O, predicting outcomes prior to the start of treatment is an art of what if's. That said, Doctor O. confirmed the concept that there are certain things patients can do to improve their outcome. What most cancer patients do not realize is the importance of exercise. Before we explore the impact of exercise on cancer let's first take a look at a plethora of health benefits associated with exercise.

Benefits of Regular Exercise

1. Reduces stress and provides a sense of balance in life.
2. Stimulates digestive enzymes and helps to reduce acid reflux.
3. Stimulates digestion and the expulsion of toxins.
4. Reduces the chance of chronic constipation and the reabsorption of toxins back into the blood.
5. Stimulates the kidney to filter higher volumes of blood.
6. Expels carbon dioxide through exhaling.
7. Purges toxins through sweat.
8. Oxygenates the brain and lungs, and improves cellular respiration throughout the entire body.
9. Maintains healthy muscles, bones and joints.
10. Purges the body of inflammation.
11. Stimulates the lymphatic system, which delivers antibodies in the form of anti-toxin lymphocytes to every area of the body.
12. Stimulates appetite.
13. Helps us sleep better.
14. Improves mental acuity.
15. Reduces incidence of heart disease and stroke.
16. Prevents and helps manage weight gain and obesity.
17. Aids in recovery from surgery.

Exercise and Cancer Prevention

The American Cancer Society (ACS), the Centers for Disease Control and Prevention (CDCP), the National Cancer Institute (NCI), the American Institute for Cancer Research (AICR), and other organizations have promoted the mental and physical health benefits of exercise for years, in particular, the important role it has in the prevention of cancer. The sweet spot for how much exercise one needs to shoot for is at least 150 minutes of moderate-intensity aerobic activity a week, ideally 30-minute periods, five days a week, or at least 75 minutes of vigorous-intensity exercise.[1]

Numerous studies indicate regular aerobic exercise is associated with a reduction in the incidence of colon, breast, lung, and endometrial cancer, in most cases by 20 percent.[2] Obesity is a well-know causative factor in many cancers, making weight management through exercise a powerful preventive mechanism. According to Professor Basen-Engquist at the University of Texas, MD Anderson, "Regular exercise can prevent obesity, which is associated with many types of cancer."[3] Studies done on colon and breast cancer patients indicate that regular aerobic exercise lessens cancer treatment induced fatigue, reduces recurrence, and improves survivability.

Cancer Treatment and Exercise

Radiation therapy kills cancer cells, but it also destroys billions of healthy cells in the targeted area, and can produce a secondary cancer down the road. It also causes burns, swelling, pain, and like chemotherapy, it can cause loss of appetite, nausea, and vomiting. This places a huge burden on the body to repair damaged cells, identify and filter out dead cells and produce new ones. The acidic burden on the body is also high. These injuries usually produce another difficult side effect, extreme fatigue. Chemotherapy is equally damaging to the body. Chemotherapeutic drugs go after rapidly growing cancer cells. Many other cells in the body also grow at a rapid pace and can be destroyed by chemo too, namely cells in the bone marrow, blood, mouth, lining of the stomach, intestine, hair, nails, and nerve endings in the hands, feet, vagina and nose. The liver and other organs can also be seriously damaged. In advanced cancer, some patients will actually die from liver failure and not the cancer itself. There are many other side effects of chemo and radiation, which will be discussed more in Chapter 13.

In years past, patients were instructed to rest during therapy and eat well. The topic of exercise never really came up. This is no longer the case. The word is getting out that exercise during cancer treatment is a proven method to help reduce the severity of side effects, particularly nausea, lack of appetite, and fatigue. So maybe it's time to put on the Under Armour, lace up the Nikes, and get the feet moving.

For most of us, the idea that exercise can reduce fatigue in cancer patients during treatment is rather counterintuitive. Yet, here is plenty of evidence to prove it does.

First, exercise stimulates a number of functions in the body. Principal among them is increased circulation of blood. Exercise activates red blood cells to carry increased amounts of oxygen and critical nutrients to cells in the body, while also increasing the export of toxins to organs that expel these toxins. Exercise stimulates the lymphatic system and white blood cells to kill pathogens. I like to think of white blood cells as being like the little curmudgeons on the Pac Man video game of years ago, where they wheel around a maze and gobble up everything they encounter—in our case the pathogens.

Second, exercise forces us to breathe in more oxygen, one of the most critical functions of life. Normal cells use oxygen for cell division. By simply increasing the level of oxygen in the blood we aid normal cell grow. Many cancer centers promote breathing exercises, five to six times a day during cancer treatment, to help the body cope with the tremendous loss of normal cells, reduce the side effects and stimulate the immune function. Of note, some alternative cancer treatment centers have reported success in treating cancer patients with pure oxygen (inhaled), intravenous hydrogen peroxide and even ozone therapy.

Now that we understand some of the science behind the ill effects of chemo and radiation and how exercise can mitigate these effects, lets take a look at a prominent research-based study.

Meta Study On Exercise

In one Meta study, in which statistical analysis is used to integrate data from a number of independent studies, researchers examined over 56 previous studies on the effect of exercise on cancer treatment related fatigue and their findings were enlightening. These previous studies covered predominately breast and prostate cancer survivors. They found that aerobic exercise significantly reduced fatigue in both breast cancer and prostate patients, but other forms of exercise, such as weight training and stretching, failed to produce the same results.[4] This does not mean that there is no value in weight training and stretching, only that it was not detected in the methodology used in this study. Researchers found that exercise significantly reduces fatigue. It also mitigates muscle wasting and severe weight loss when bedridden.

They also promoted the idea that exercise should be added to follow up treatment plans to produce the greatest benefit from the treatment. The other interventions recommended were counseling in the areas of mental health, nutrition, stress management, and sleep therapy.[5]

It is easy to extend the benefits of exercise from this study to most other cancers. I am convinced it played a significant role in my recovery and so did my oncology team. During treatment, I met with Doctor O. every week and he always inquired as to how well I was eating, sleeping, and exercising. He explained,

> Joe, the chemo and radiation will wear you out more as each week passes. Patients normally lose a lot of weight and experience difficulty eating, and you will not be able to exercise at the same level as treatment progresses. It would be fantastic if you continue jogging or take walks every a day.

During our week four visit he was amazed that I had only lost a couple of pounds and that I was still doing cardio. Others are much less fortunate than I was. For example, they might enter treatment with other health issues, or with a compromised immune system that prohibits them from even walking. It is critical for those in this situation to speak with their doctor, or an exercise physiologist, or some other expert to help them find activities that can get their body active and moving again. It is surprising how many exercises are possible by staying in one spot, such as Yoga and Pilates. Patients can also get some exercise by doing simple dance or martial arts movements while sitting or standing in one spot.

The oncology team gave me a number of range-of-motion exercises I could do sitting, standing, or laying in bed. They also gave me simple resistance exercises I could do while leaning against a wall. Talk to your cancer team and let them help you learn how to use exercise to recover from treatment quickly.

So what level of intensity of exercise should those in cancer treatment shoot for? Most experts recommend moderate-intensity activities at least five days a week for a minimum of 30 minutes. Research also shows a strong inverse relationship with the amount of exercise and the impact on survival rates, particularly for those with colon cancer. In other words, the more vigorous the exercise, the higher the survival rate. These activities can include brisk walks, jogging, and any other type of exercise that gets your heart rate up to a moderate level.[6] In terms of setting goals, monitoring progress, and in providing feedback to your doctor, it is beneficial to understand some terminology and how intensity levels are distinguished. Whatever level you find yourself in, set a goal to inch your way up the ladder to the next higher level. Now it's time to examine the difference between low, moderate and vigorous exercise.

Levels of Exercise

Low Intensity: An activity that raises heart rate up to 30% to 54% of maximum for your age group. Examples include:
– Walking at a rate of 2 to 3 miles per hour (MPH).
– Riding a bicycle at 10 MPH.
– A 2 MPH pace equals a 30-minute mile.
– A 3 MPH pace equals a 20-minute mile.
– A 10 MPH pace equals a 6-minute mile.
Moderate Intensity: An activity that raises heart rate up to 55% to 70% of maximum heart rate. Examples include walking at 3 to 5 MPH, or 20-minute miles, or bicycling at 10 to 20 MPH.
Vigorous Intensity: An activity that raises heart rate up to 70% to 95% of maximum heart rate. Examples of this include running at 5 MPH or faster, or bicycling at a speed greater than 20 MPH.[7]

There are many other activities that can substitute for running or bicycling. The important thing is to pick something you enjoy doing and stick with it.

Another method to measure exercise intensity is to monitor heart rate. This is an excellent approach since it provides instantaneous biofeedback and allows one to monitor their progress and make adjustments on the run, so to speak. All you need is a heart rate monitor that you can strap to your wrist or chest. Some watches have built in heart rate sensors and these sensors are also found on various cardio machines at the fitness center.

There is great gratification in being able to get into a routine and monitor your heart rate each time you exercise, and then watch yourself make progress. Now it's time to look at how exercise intensity is determined using heart rate.

Exercise Intensity

The most popular formula used to measure exercise intensity using heart rate takes age and subtracts it from 220. This number identifies the heart rate for the maximum level of intensity for your age. The American Heart Association and many other health organizations use this formula as their figure of merit for exercise intensity. Here is an example: If you are 50 years old, subtract 50 from 220 and you get a maximum heart rate of 170 beats per minute (BPM). The heart rate for each level of intensity is defined by the following percentages of the maximum BPM:

Low: 50 to 70 percent of maximum heart rate at 170 BPM
Moderate: 71 to 85 percent of maximum heart rate at 170 BPM
High: 86 to 100 percent of maximum heart rate at 170 BPM

Using the above formula, three levels of intensity can then be segmented into age groups according to a predetermined factor that accounts for reduced cardio vascular function.

Age	Low Intensity	Moderate Intensity	Max Intensity
20	100-170	171-199	200
30	95-162	163-189	90
35	93-157	158-184	185
40	90-153	154-179	180
45	88-149	150-174	175
50	85-145	146-169	170
55	83-140	141-164	165
60	80-136	137-159	160
65	78-132	133-154	155
70	75-128	129-149	150

As cancer treatment progresses, it takes more and more out of the patient and the harder it becomes to get out of bed each day. By the end of treatment many of us are so overcome with fatigue we don't want to get out of bed. Consigning ourselves to bed has all sorts of ill effects, including severe weight loss, weakened joints and muscles, constipation, breathing problems, skin sores, emotional changes, and depression. Radiation treatment to the esophagus is so painful most have difficulty swallowing by the fourth week of treatment and are forced to go on a liquid diet. I was one of the more fortunate ones and was able to swallow whole food all the way through five weeks of radiation. All of my doctors and nurses were amazed at this too. My Radiation Oncologist was shocked when he was not able to find a single radiation burn on my back or stomach throughout the entire treatment period. Exercise played a huge role in this outcome. I also have to give credit to an alkaline diet and targeted natural substances, which are discussed in the next chapter.

Post Treatment Exercise

Experiencing a recurrence of cancer is a devastating experience. Therefore, understanding the role of exercise in helping prevent recurrence is worth its weight in gold. During a post treatment surveillance examination, about four weeks after treatment, I asked Doctor O., "How big a factor is vigorous exercise in helping prevent recurrence?" He replied, "Exercise, along with a balanced diet, are probably the two most important things you can do to help recover from treatment and prevent recurrence."

Other Studies on Exercise

In one key study that examined the effect of exercise on preventing recurrence, researchers added two other variables known to have a cancer preventive benefit. In addition to exercise, they required the control group to maintain a body mass index (BMI) of 25 kg/m or less, and to not drink more than one alcoholic drink a day.

A BMI greater than 25 indicates someone is overweight. Previous studies also showed women who drank no more than one alcoholic drink a day, and men who drank no more than two alcoholic drinks a day, experienced a cancer prevention benefit. In this study however, researchers only examined women.

They identified 2,905 women from a high risk Breast Cancer Family Register in New York. Seventy-seven percent of these women were Caucasian and 23 percent Hispanic. They recorded a mortality of 312, with an average survival of 9.1 years following treatment. The survivability results of this study are phenomenal.

Women who adhered to the cancer prevention protocol were associated with a stunning 44 to 53 percent lower incidence of mortality than those who did not. The range of numbers in their statistics is there because they stratified the data into different groups according to age, race, and two risk categories: BRCA1 and BRAC2 carriers. Amazingly, the association with lower mortality remained relatively intact across all groups.[8]

I don't know about you, but when I read this study I could not help but imagine what the impact might be if this study added four more control variables, sugar avoidance, a balanced alkaline diet, a low stress job, and no tobacco use.

Another large study examined close to 3,000 women with non-metastatic breast cancer. They discovered that women who engaged in the equivalent of walking three to five hours per week at a moderate pace, were significantly less likely to die from breast cancer, than those who did not exercise at this level.[9]

In another observational study, conducted in 2014, researchers evaluated the effect of exercise on a group of over 1,000 men diagnosed with a range of cancers. Their findings were not surprising. Men who performed the most vigorous and frequent physical exercise had the highest survival rate, compared to those who performed less exercise. The level of exercise was estimated as equivalent to 45 to 60 minutes of hiking or jogging five days a week.[10]

Summary

Research on exercise and cancer is loud and clear. Those who exercise regularly gain a significant benefit in resisting cancer, tolerating cancer treatment, recovering from treatment faster, and in preventing recurrence, compared to those who do not exercise. It also shows a strong direct relationship with the amount of exercise and its impact on survival rates. That is to say, the more vigorous one exercises the higher their rate of survival.

If exercising daily is a new habit for you, then build a routine slowly. If you encounter obstacles that block your progress, do not become discouraged. It is a gauntlet we all walk through. One can always find a way around an obstacle blocking their path. If you find yourself wanting to quit, then be persistent and do not give up. Persistence is the calisthenics of success. As the great football coach Vince Lombardi once said, "The harder you work, the harder it is to quit." If you are undergoing cancer treatment, then force yourself to get out of bed to take a walk or do a resistance exercise against a wall, because everything we do to help our situation matters. If you make progress, then treat yourself and eat something yummy you haven't had in a while. In the end however, there is a reward greater than any other—and that is, the satisfaction gained from accomplishing something that is otherwise difficult to achieve, even in its slightest form. This is about the sweetest treat of them all. As far as cancer patients and exercise go, there is only one road to take. Just do it!

Notes

1. "Fitting in Fitness", The American Cancer Society. http://www. can cer.org/healthy/eathealthy getactive/getactive/fitting-in-fitness (accessed November 2, 2015).

2. The National Cancer Institute and the National Institute of Health, "Physical Activity and Cancer", http://www.cancer.gov/about-cancer/causes-prevention/risk/obesity/physical-activity-fact-sheet (accessed January 22, 2015).

3. "Exercise and Cancer Prevention: Benefits of Exercise Apply to a Variety of Cancers", OncoLog, July 2012, Vol. 57, No. 7, 1.

4. "The Effect of Exercise on Cancer Related Fatigue." News Author Kate Johnson, CME Author Hien T. Nghiem, MD Faculty and Disclosures, CME Released 12/14/2014. Medscape Multispecialty; http://www.medscape.org/viewarticle/775325
(accessed October 9, 2015, 1-3).

5. Ibid.

6. Ibid.

7. "The Role of Physical Activity in Cancer Prevention, Treatment, Recovery, and Survivorship", ONCOLOGY, Review Article 1 June, 2013, by Dawn Lemanne, MD, MPH, Barrie R. Cassileth, MS, PhD, and Jyorthirmai Gubili, MS, http://www.cancernetwork.com/survivorship /role-physical-activity-cancer-prevention-treatment-recovery-and-survivorship (accessed October 9, 2015).

8. Cloud AJ, Thai A, Liao Y, Terry MB. The impact of cancer prevention guideline adherence on overall mortality in a high-risk cohort of women from the New York site of the Breast Cancer Family Registry. Breast Cancer Res Treat. 2015;149:537-546.
http://www.medscape.com/medline/abstract/25604794 (accessed October 9, 2015).

9. Holmes MD, et al., "Physical Activity and Survival After Breast Cancer Diagnosis." JAMA, 2005:293:2479-2486. Abstract.

10. Mythbusters: Complementary and Alternative Treatments in Cancer, Victoria Stern, MA, September 02, 2014; http://www.topsfield-ma.gov /health/documents/MythbustersComplementaryandAlternative TreatmentsinCancer.pdf (accessed 9/14/2014, 8).

CHAPTER 11

Natural Supplements And Cancer

By the river on its bank will grow all kinds of trees for food . . . and their leaves will be for healing.
—Ezekiel 47:12

In the ninth chapter of the Gospel of John, in the New Testament of the Bible, Jesus healed a man who was blind from birth in a peculiar manner. Although there are a number of messages in this passage, I will only explore the method he used to heal. Jesus spat on the ground and formed a paste with his saliva and the dirt. He applied the mud to the blind man's eyes and instructed him to go to the pool of Siloam and wash it off. The blind man obeyed and was miraculously healed. Jesus could have used his supernatural powers to heal him instantly, but he didn't. So, why did Jesus use this method? Some might say that the pool of Siloam was used for ritualistic cleansing of the priests who served in the Temple and that washing there was symbolic of the washing away of sin; but no one really knows for sure. Perhaps Jesus knew that there were certain minerals in the dirt that when mixed with the enzymes in his spit would create a healing ointment. Who would better know the chemistry of everything in the natural world than the Creator Himself? It makes me wonder if Jesus used this method as a master pharmacist would, taking the things of nature and forming them into a perfect healing salve. Such perfect knowledge is beyond our grasp. Yet, we do not need perfect knowledge to defeat cancer, we only need just enough.

There exists substantial scientific knowledge in regard to natural substances that fight cancer, which is the topic of this chapter.

Cancer patients who provide their bodies with the highest level of nutritional support will resist infections, tolerate chemo and radiation better, experience fewer post-treatment complications and recover faster. A stronger post-treatment immune system will also help the body tolerate any follow-on treatments and resist recurrence, ultimately producing better outcomes.

Yet, controversy exists over taking high doses of antioxidants, which are well-known anticancer agents, while undergoing chemotherapy. Antioxidants are nutrients that trigger the body's immune system to seek out and destroy pathogens. They include Vitamins A, C, E, Selenium, Zinc, and carotenes, such as Lycopene, found in tomatoes and Beta-carotene, found in carrots. Some studies suggest high doses of antioxidants make chemo-radiation less effective because they provide cancer cells extra strength to resist the therapy. Other studies indicate the opposite, especially when the vitamins are in the foods we eat. Supporters of antioxidants claim that prior research is flawed because it only looked at high doses of a single antioxidant, and that when a diet is rich in a broad range of antioxidants, they partner with each other and are more effective.[1]

For those who like to know the what, why and how behind the things we ingest for health reasons, there is nothing more important than having a relevant and accurate piece of literature to read. Unfortunately, the Internet is loaded with excessive amounts of information on supplements. Sorting through all of this information and making sense of it for your type of cancer is overwhelming and extremely time consuming. This chapter provides a synopsis of some key supplements that have cancer-fighting qualities and are backed up by scientific research and numerous doctors.

So which supplements should one take? It depends. Let's look at some of the most highly touted supplements by alternative, integrative and naturopathic doctors.

The supplements in this list have all been extensively studied in the laboratory and in observational human studies as being safe to take and effective in helping the body fight cancer. Most of these supplements are also highly recommended by naturopathic doctors at the Cancer Treatment Centers of America.

Top Supplements

1. Vitamin C
2. Selenium
3. Vitamin D3
4. Pancreatic Enzymes
5. Curcumin or Quercetin
6. Maitake Mushroom MD Fraction
7. Green Tea Extract
8. Melatonin
9. Modified Citrus Pectin
10. CoQ10

The dosages sited are ones that Naturopathic Doctors recommended to me. For more information on therapeutic dosages that pertain to your situation please consult with a Naturopathic Doctor, or the book, *How to Prevent and Treat Cancer with Natural Medicine.*

1. Vitamin C. Dosage: 5,000 to 10, 000 mg (5-10 g) per day. Vitamin C is one of the most well documented immune system support vitamins ever studied and is extremely safe to take at high doses. A common side effect of taking too much Vitamin C is diarrhea. Some recommend a dosage two to three times the dose I take because they strongly believe in Vitamin C's ability to fight cancer. Intravenous (IV) Vitamin C is also offered by a number of alternative cancer centers. High dose IV Vitamin C is proven to be safe, but still needs to be done under the supervision of a doctor.

2. Selenium. Dosage: 400 mcg (or 0.4 mg) per day. Selenium is an essential mineral in the body and works as a powerful antioxidant, especially when used with Vitamin E. Selenium greatly reinforces the immune system by stimulating white blood cell activity and numerous studies show it exhibits significant anti-cancer qualities. In one study, those who took selenium showed a 50 percent reduced risk of dying from numerous types of cancer.[2]

In a multi-year study published in 1996 by the American Medical Association, which included over 1,300 patients the powerful cancer prevention qualities of selenium were established. Patients were given 200 mcg of selenium a day over a 4.5-year period. This study covered multiple cancer centers and was double blind, randomized and placebo-controlled. Researchers reported a 51 percent reduction in total cancer mortality and over a 40 percent reduction in prostrate cancer. Consult with a doctor before taking more than the daily-recommended level of selenium because it can be extremely toxic if taken in high doses.

3. Vitamin D3. Dosage: 5,000 or more IU per day. Absorption is improved if taken sublingually in a micellized form. Vitamin D3 is classified as both a vitamin and a hormone and performs numerous helpful functions throughout the body. Vitamin D is synthesized in the body from vitamin D3 taken orally, or through exposure to ultraviolet rays from sunlight. It plays a key role in the absorption of calcium. To increase the absorption of D3 it should be taken sublingually as micellized D3 with Vitamin K2.

Vitamin D3 can stimulates mechanisms in the immune system to prevent, reduce progression, and inhibit the recurrence of cancer. In a study done by the University of California, San Diego School of Medicine, researchers discovered that breast cancer patients with high levels of vitamin D in their blood are twice as likely to survive their disease as women with low levels of this nutrient.[3] Other research shows that an overwhelming number of women who get breast cancer are significantly deficient in Vitamin D.

4. Pancreatic Enzymes. Dosage: Pancreatin 4X, 400 mg, three times per day. Also known as Proteolytic Enzymes; they are derived from pig enzymes. Biotics Research Corporation manufactures them under the label Intenzyme Forte. They are enteric-coated to prevent digestion prior to entering the small intestine and should be taken on an empty stomach. A number of other substances are in these supplements that assist in stimulating enzyme activity, digestion and absorption. The main ingredient is Pancreatin and comes in various concentrations, such as 4X or 8X, meaning four or eight times the standard concentration.

Pancreatin falls under the category of enzyme therapy and became a popular treatment used by alternative practitioners in the early 20th century. In recent years, Doctor Nicholas Gonzalez popularized it. He used pancreatic enzymes successfully in high dose therapy for advanced pancreatic cancer patients. Doctor Gonzalez recently passed, but his treatment center in New York City continues his work. Pancreatic enzymes are widely accepted by numerous naturopathic doctors as a credible anticancer fighting agent as well as a safe supplement to take during chemo, radiation and surgery.

Clinical studies suggest that pancreatic enzymes increase life expectancy in numerous types of cancer and it also helps reduce the horrible side effects of chemo and radiation therapy. Studies indicate that pancreatic enzymes reduce the side effects of chemo and radiation, and the rate of treatment induced viral infections. Pancreatic enzymes are believed to breakdown the outer walls of cancer cells and make them more susceptible to chemotherapy, nutritional therapy, natural substance therapy and fasting. There is a caution to not take these enzymes for at least three days prior to or following surgery, because they may increase the risk of bleeding.[4]

Supporters of pancreatic enzymes claim there is established clinical and observational evidence that suggests they not only inhibit progression of disease for most cancers, but they also improve outcomes. To their credit, numerous scientific and medical studies support their claims.

Doctor Michael Murray is a world renowned Naturopathic Doctor and is a huge advocate of these enzymes for treating cancer. For more info go to http://www.DoctorMurray.com.[5] He also coauthored an extensively documented book, *How To Prevent And Treat Cancer With Natural Medicine*, with a number of other naturopathic doctors.

5. Curcumin. Dosage: 3 to 5 grams, one to two times a day. Some doctors suggest doses as high as 10 to 12 grams per day. High does of curcumin can create serious gastric discomfort. The biggest obstacle of getting the anticancer benefit of curcumin is that very little of it is absorbed into the body during digestion. Several supplement companies combine certain enzymes with curcumin to increase absorption. Curcu Gel Ultra is a brand highly recommended by Consumer Labs that great increases bioavailability.

Curcumin is a substance found in the Indian spices turmeric and curry. The side effects of curcumin are similar to those of eating too much spicy food, such as flatulence, indigestion and nausea. Long-term use can also lead to stomach ulcers and other problems, according to the American Cancer Society.[6] Curcumin should not be taken on an empty stomach.

Curcumin is considered an antioxidant with numerous studies indicating it has strong anticancer mechanisms, especially in colon cancer. In animal studies, curcumin not only reduces the risk of colon cancer but also inhibits progression in all stages, and inhibits recurrence after treatment.[7] As an antioxidant, it is shown to be as much as 300 times more effective than Vitamin E.[8] It is also a strong anti-inflammatory agent. Numerous studies with animals and human cancer cells indicate curcumin is a powerful agent in cleansing the body of carcinogens and in enhancing production of glutathione, the most powerful antioxidant in the body. One study suggested curcumin suppressed tumor growth by inhibiting epidermal growth factor receptor sites on cancer cells.[9] In a study published by the National Institute of Health, researchers said,

> Our review shows that curcumin can kill a wide variety of tumor cell types through diverse mechanisms. Because of numerous mechanisms of cell death employed by curcumin, it is possible that cells may not develop resistance to curcumin induced cell death. Furthermore, its ability to kill tumor cells and not normal cells makes curcumin an attractive candidate for drug development. Although numerous animal studies and clinical trials have been done, additional studies are needed to gain the full benefit from curcumin.[10]

In another study published in the Journal of Breast Cancer, researchers summarized how curcumin acts as an antitumor agent in breast cancer cells. They sited studies where portions of human breast cancer tumors were implanted into animals and curcumin prohibited their progression. They pointed out that curcumin is not water-soluble and this contributes to low bioavailability, meaning it is difficult for it to be transported throughout the body's aqueous environment and cell structure. They proposed more study on synthetic delivery agents or nano-technology based formulas as delivery agents.[11]

Despite a plethora of research that shows the anticancer effects of curcumin, some traditional oncologists and organizations are not convinced. Case in point: Mayo Clinic states that there is insufficient evidence to recommend curcumin as a cancer fighting substance.[12] Nonetheless, other research indicates curcumin can help reduce the side effects of chemo and radiation and can be safely taken while undergoing treatment.[13]

A substance that is strikingly similar to curcumin is **quercetin**. It is well known for its anti-inflammatory and anticancer chemical agents and can be used instead of curcumin if curcumin is not well tolerated. Quercetin is found in green tea, apples, onions and white grapefruit and has a powerful ability to inhibit tumor formation by preventing cancer cells from dividing.[14]

6. Maitake Mushrooms – MD Fraction. The recommended dosage is 1 mg for every two pounds of body weight.[15] Natural Factors Maitake Gold 404 is an excellent brand and it also comes in a sublingual tincture, which can help increase absorption.

Using Maitake mushrooms to fight cancer has a long history in Chinese and Japanese medicine. The West has been slow to catch on. A number of substances in Maitake mushrooms have a proven ability to bolster the immune system, prevent cancer, and inhibit its progression. In particular, it protects healthy cells—it stimulates white blood cells to seek out and destroy cancer cells—it increases programmed cell death——and it inhibits progression of cancer.[16] Some researchers combined Maitake with traditional chemotherapy and found that it increased five-year disease-free survival (DFS) by 12 percent in stomach cancer patients. When it was added to radiation treatment in Non-Small Cell Lung Cancer (NSCLC) it increased survival by 39 percent for Stage 1 and 2 patients, and by 22 percent for Stage 3 patients.[17] Following are additional studies that support the use of Maitake mushroom extract as a safe complement to fighting cancer.

A study published by the NIH in 2011 stated, "Maitake (D fraction) mushroom extract induces apoptosis [cell death] in breast cancer cells by BAK-1 gene activation."[18]

Researchers from Memorial Sloan Kettering Cancer Center, in collaboration with The New York Presbyterian Hospital Weill Medical College of Cornell University, concluded that Maitake mushroom extract can reduce the growth of cancer in animals by activating their white blood cells; however, there is no evidence that it can kill cancer cells directly.[19]

In a study published by the International Journal of General Medicine, researchers summarized numerous studies that have been

151

performed in the laboratory, in animals and in humans using Maitake mushroom, and concluded,

> These studies showed that PDF [the active substance in Maitake] was indeed capable of modulating immunologic and hematologic parameters, inhibiting or regressing the cancer cell growth, and even improving quality of life of cancer patients.[20]

They further stated that there is evidence from human studies that using Maitake and intravenous Vitamin C has great potential as a combination therapy against cancer.

7. <u>Green Tea Extract</u>. Dosage: 500 mg, one per day. According to the NCI, Green Tea must be taken cautiously because there are numerous potential side effects, including gas, nausea, heartburn, stomach ache, abdominal pain, dizziness, headache and muscle pain.[21] Green Tea might also contain high levels of caffeine. Start with a low dose of it and test for tolerance before taking a high dose.

The flavonoids and polyphenols found in Green Tea are well researched and proven to have excellent anticancer properties. Flavonoids are also known for their anti-inflammatory, antiviral and anti-allergic effects. Flavonoids are also found in quercetin. Taking Green Tea extract however, provides a much greater concentration of flavonoids than can be achieved through food. Green Tea extract is safely used with conventional chemotherapy.[22]

According to the NCI, Green tea is the most studied of all teas. In animal studies the polyphenols are found to inhibit tumor growth in skin, lung, oral, esophagus, stomach, small intestine, colon, liver, pancreas, and mammary gland cancer. However, in human studies the results are inconclusive, probably due to variables such as differences in tea preparation and consumption, the variances in the type of tea studied, and the bioavailability of the tea compounds, along with other factors. Few trials have examined the effects of green tea on the incidence of cancer or mortality.[23]

8. <u>Melatonin</u>. Dosage: 20 mg per day, best taken before bed each night. Some therapeutic doses are as high as 40 mg. Common side effects in are headaches, dizziness, and sleepiness, if taken during the day. This is why it is supposed to be taken before bed each night. It might also

interact with other medications, so keep your doctor informed and start with a small dose and work your way up.[24] During treatment I experienced headaches after taking 20 mg per night for three weeks and reduced the dose down to 3 to 5 mg.

Melatonin is a hormone in the body, which supports the endocrine system. Its primary function is to regulate sleep-wake cycles, and it can be an excellent sleep aid. A number of studies strongly suggest melatonin has anti-tumoral effects and improves survival in cancer patients. According to one study, "Taking high doses of melatonin with chemotherapy or other cancer treatments might reduce tumor size and improve survival rates in people with tumors."[25]

In one clinical study, 30 node-relapsed melanoma patients who had completed chemotherapy were randomized to receive no treatment, or 20 mg of melatonin orally in the evening.

> After a median follow-up of 31 months, the percent of DFS [disease free survival] was significantly higher in melatonin-treated individuals than in controls. The DFS curve was also significantly longer in the melatonin group than in controls. No melatonin related toxicity was observed.[26]

This study indicates that melatonin is effective at inhibiting progression of node relapsed melanoma patients. Other research indicates melatonin can enhance the effectiveness of chemo and radiation therapy. It is believed that melatonin may stimulate the P53 gene, which is a gene that can cause cancer cell suicide.[27]

> Studies have shown that patients taking melatonin (20 mg a day) had significantly less weight loss (3 kg vs. 16 kg) and a lower chance of disease progression (53 percent vs. 90 percent) compared with those treated with supportive care.[28]

In a study of chemotherapy versus chemo-endocrine therapy as a first line of treatment for NSCLC patients, the outcomes were substantially better for the chemo-endocrine therapy patients. One-year survival was significantly higher in patients treated with melatonin plus chemotherapy (15 out of 34), compared to those who received chemotherapy alone (7 out of 36). Of note, one of the melatonin patients experienced a complete response, meaning the cancer went into remission. Patients who received melatonin also tolerated the chemo side effects much better than those who did not. Specifically, the frequency of bone marrow suppression, neuropathy, and cachexia was significantly lower in the melatonin group. This study shows that melatonin may improve the efficacy of chemotherapy and reduce toxicity in patients in poor clinical condition.[29]

9. <u>Modified Citrus Pectin</u> (MCP). Dosage: 3 to 5 grams, three times a day. Some doctors recommend doses as high as 15 grams per day. Growing evidence suggests that MCP has powerful cancer fighting mechanisms. In one study, researchers concluded that MCP inhibits cancer cells from combining to form tumors in areas of the body outside the primary tumor, and causing some cancer cells to commit cell suicide.[30] MCP demonstrates characteristics that may even prevent cancer cells from forming into a tumor in the first place. "MCP has been shown to be effective either against prostate carcinoma, colon carcinoma, breast carcinoma, melanoma, multiple myeloma, and hemangiosarcoma [canine blood vessel cancer]."[31] These same researchers argue that even though there are limited studies on humans, one human study of MCP indicated that it significantly inhibited the progression of prostate cancer and doubled the survival time of recurrent prostate cancer patients.[32]

At an American Chemical Society Symposium, Doctor Isaac Eliaz presented an extensive summary on the anticancer mechanisms of MCP. Most notably, he pointed out that there exists substantial scientific evidence that MCP prevents angiogenesis, which means it blocks the ability of cancer cells to form new blood vessels. MCP also helps remove heavy metals from the body without affecting essential minerals.[33] MCP has emerged as an extremely promising substance that can inhibit cancer cells from forming into tumors and also prevent its spread to other areas of the body.

10. <u>CoQ10</u>: Dosage: 300 to 400 mg per day, taken at intervals. CoQ10 is a substance that profits many areas of the body. It contains strong antioxidant properties and is found in all cells. CoQ10 aids the heart, energy levels, cognition, helps in treating macular degeneration, Alzheimer's, migraine headaches, chronic fatigue syndrome and it is an important agent in a cell's ability to produce ATP, the energy needed for cell growth. CoQ10 also exhibits anti-cancer properties. Ubiquinol

is considered the most effective form CoQ10. The sublingual and liquid forms are the most absorbable.

According to the National Cancer Institute, lower CoQ10 levels are frequently found in those with cancer as compared to those without cancer. As an anticancer agent, CoQ10 has been shown to enhance the effects of both conventional and alternative therapy. Some studies indicate noticeable anticancer benefit when CoQ10 is used with other antioxidants, such as Vitamin C, Selenium, folic acid and beta-carotenes. In other studies going back 20 years, CoQ10 caused complete remission in some early stage breast cancer patients, and demonstrated significant anticancer effects with prostrate cancer.

Summary

This chapter examined a number of natural supplements that exhibit significant immune boosting and anticancer qualities that can be safely used as a complement to any type of treatment program. Many of these supplements can also reduce the debilitating side effects of chemo and radiation, and in some cases they can even enhance the effectiveness of chemotherapy. All of these natural supplements are readily available, scientifically supported and safe to use.

One of the most significant things I learned in regard to natural supplements is buyer beware. This is a poorly regulated industry and there are numerous products that may not contain anything close to the substances they are advertising. It is extremely important to consult with objective and credible testing and reviews, such as those produced by Consumer Labs, before throwing money at something. An Internet subscription to Consumer Labs is only about 30 dollars a year and the information they provide is well worth every penny. Cancer patients cannot afford to waste time with a substandard supplement. Cutting corners on price will usually result in an inferior product.

Everything we do to fight cancer contributes to how long we might survive. Taking vitamins and supplements that are proven to support the immune system, prevent cancer, slow progression, prevent recurrence, and reduce the side effects of treatment, can be one of those game changers. However, if we do not reinforce our body with a well-balanced alkaline diet, daily exercise, a positive emotional and mental state, and a low-stress life situation, the positive effects of any supplements will be greatly diminished.

I hope my research and testimony saves you valuable time, decreases your anxiety, and encourages you to believe that the patient can make a tremendous difference in their healing outcome.

God has the power to supernaturally heal us—yet one might suspect that he more frequently operates at the cellular level through the laws of biology, chemistry and physics that he created. Therefore, any extra wisdom or knowledge we gain in how to help our body heal from cancer might make the difference as to whether we visit the pool of Siloam, or some other pool.

Notes

1. Murray, Michael, ND, Birdsall, Tim, ND, Pizzorno, Joseph E. ND, Reilly, Paul, ND, *How to Prevent and Treat Cancer with Natural Medicine*, Endorsed by the Cancer Treatment Centers of America. (New York: Riverhead Books), 2002, 53 - 55.
2. Ibid., 56 - 57.
3. "Vitamin D Increases Breast Cancer Patient Survival," University of California, San Diego School of Medicine, Anticancer Research, March 06, 2014, http://health.ucsd.edu/news/releases/Pages/2014-03 -06-vitamin-D-and-breast-cancer-survival.aspx (accessed December 7, 2015).
4. "How to Prevent and Treat Cancer . . . ," 168 -171.
5. "Healing Power of Proteolytic Enzymes." Doctor Michael Murray, ND. http://doctormurray.com/tag/proteolytic-enzymes/ (accessed December 7, 2015, 1-20).
6. Lee, Jill, "Side Effects of the Curcumin in Turmeric", Updated: Apr 16, 2015, //www.livestrong.com/article/112941-side-effects-turmeric curcumin (accessed December 4, 2015).
7 Ibid., 102.
8. "How to Prevent and Treat Cancer . . . ," 72.
9. Ibid.,174-175.
10. Ravindran, Jayaraj et al, "Curcumin and Cancer Cells: How Many Ways Can Curry Kill Tumor Cells Selectively?" AAPS Journal 2009 Sep; 11(3):495–510. Published online 2009 Jul 10, http://www.ncbi.nlm.nih.gov/pmc/articles/PMC2758121 (accessed December 3, 2015).
11. Dongwu Liu and Zhiwei Chen, "The Effect of Curcumin on Breast Cancer Cells", Journal of Breast Cancer, 2014 Jun; 16(2) 133-137.
12. Moynihan, Timothy J. M.D., "Can Curcumin Slow Cancer Growth?", http://www.mayoclinic.org/diseases-conditions/cancer/expert-answers/curcumin/FAQ-20057858 (accessed December 3, 2015).
13. "How to Prevent and Treat Cancer . . . ," 241-242.
14. Ibid., 72, 176.
15. Ibid., 240.
16. Ibid., 177-179,
17. Ibid., 240-241.
18. Soares, R. et al., "Maitake (D fraction) Mushroom Extract Induces Apoptosis in Breast Cancer Cells by BAK-1 Gene Activation." J Med Food. 2011 Jun;14(6):563-72. doi: 10.1089/jmf.2010.0095. Epub

2011Apr 11. Abstract, http://www.ncbi.nlm.nih.gov/pubmed/21480800 (accessed December 8, 2015).

19. "Does Maitake Mushroom Extract Enhance Hematopoiesis in Myelo dysplastic Patients?" Sponsored by Memorial Sloan Kettering Cancer Center, ClinicalTrials.gov Identifier: NCT01099917, April 5, 2010, https://clinicaltrials.gov/ct2/show/NCT01099917 (accessed December 8, 2015).

20. Konno, Sensuke, "Synergistic Potentiation of D-Fraction with Vitamin C as Possible Alternative Approach for Cancer Therapy," Abstract, International Journal of General Medicine 2009; 2: 91–108.Published online 2009 Jul 30, http://www.ncbi.nlm. nih.gov/pmc/articles/PMC2840554 (accessed December 8, 2015).

21. "Tea and Cancer Prevention: Strengths and Limits of the Evidence", National Cancer Institute. http://www.cancer.gov/about-cancer/causes-prevention/risk/diet/tea-fact -sheet (accessed December 8, 2015, 2).

22. "How to Prevent and Treat Cancer . . . ," 161.

23. "Tea and Cancer Prevention . . . ," 2, 3.

24. "Is Melatonin a Helpful Sleep Aid - and What Should I Know About Melatonin Side Effects?" Answers from Brent A. Baurer, M.D., http://www.mayoclinic.org/healthy-lifestyle/adult-health/expert-answers /melatonin -side-effects/faq-20057874 (accessed December 9, 2015).

25. "Melatonin - How Effective Is It?" MedlinePlus, U.S. National Library of Medicine. https://www.nlm.nih.gov/medlineplus/drug info/natural/ 940.html (accessed December 9, 2015).

26. Lissoni P, Brivio O, Brivio F, et al. "Adjuvant Therapy with the Pineal Hormone Melatonin in Patients with Lymph Node Relapse due to Malignant Melanoma," Abstract, Journal of Pineal Research, pages 239–242, November 1996, http://onlinelibrary.wiley.com/doi/ 10.1111/j.1600 -079X.1996.tb00292.x/abstract (accessed December 9, 2015).

27. "How to Prevent and Treat Cancer . . .," 242.

28. Ibid., 243.

29. Lissoni P, Palorossi F, et al. "A Randomized Study of Chemotherapy with Cisplatin Plus Etoposide Versus Chemoendocrine Therapy with Cisplatin, Etoposide and the Pineal Hormone Melatonin as a First-Line Treatment of Advanced Non-Small Cell Lung Cancer (NSCLC) Patients in a Poor Clinical State." Abstract, Journal of Pineal Research, Volume 23, Issue 1, pages 15-19, August 1997. http://onlinelibrary.wiley.com/doi/ 10.1111 /j.1600-079X.1997. tb00329.x/abstract (accessed December 9, 2015).

30. Vladislav V. Glinsky and Avraham Raz. "Modified Citrus Pectin Anti

-Metastatic Properties: One Bullet, Multiple Targets,"Carbohydr Res. 2009 Sep 28: 344(14): 1788-1791, Conclusions. http://www.ncbi.nlm.nih.gov/pmc/articles/PMC2782490 (accessed December 22, 2015, 5).

31. Ibid., 1.

32. Ibid., 5.

33. "American Chemical Society Highlights Modified Citrus Pectin as Solution to Chronic Disease Marker Galectin-3." Better Health Publishing, 22-Aug-2012.http://www.newswise.com/articles/american-chemical-society- highlights-modified-citrus-pectin-as-solution-to-chronic-disease-marker-galectin-3 (accessed December 22, 2015).

CHAPTER 12

Sodium Bicarbonate And Cancer

When the solution is simple, God is answering.
—Albert Einstein

D octor B., a Resident Surgeon, walked into the examination
room and introduced himself and started making small talk
with us. I was sitting on the examination table with my
notebook and pen in my lap. I was not prepared to bring up sodium
bicarbonate, so I left it off my list of questions. This was the first of
several pre-surgery meetings.

After some pleasantries, Doctor B. examined me, and then asked if I
had any questions for the surgeon. I said, "I'm really concerned about
the surgery. If the chemo and radiation are successful, and there is no
evidence of cancer, can I avoid the surgery and go on surveillance?" He
answered, "Unfortunately, the surgery is the key component of the
standard of care and we always do it unless the patient is compromised
by something else." I said, "I believe my body can heal itself if given
the right support. In fact, my tumor shrank from 4 cm to 1.5 cm prior
to entering treatment, and the Barrett's Esophagus resolved itself." He
looked surprised, then said, "That's really interesting; let me take a look
at your diagnostics again." He walked over to the desk and paged

through my records. Then he said, "For a tumor to regress is pretty unusual and I've never heard of Barrett's healing on its own. Your diagnostics seem to indicate something good is happening with you." He folded his arms and asked, "Can you tell me what you think may have caused this to happen?" His question caught me off guard. I said, "I believe it was mostly from my cancer diet, daily exercise and all the prayer I've received." However, I wasn't ready to share with him my experimentation with sodium bicarbonate. He nodded his head and smiled, placed the folder on the desk and said, "Let's see if the surgeon is ready to see you." We shook hands, and he headed for the door. As he opened the door, he looked back, and said, "Whatever you're doing, keep doing it, because it's working." Kelly and I looked at each other and smiled. He just validated the basis of my whole personal treatment plan, that the patient plays a critical role in affecting the outcome of his or her health. Are you ready for some exciting new information? Let's dive in now.

Sodium Bicarbonate

Sodium bicarbonate, otherwise known as Baking Soda, is an ancient substance used for a myriad of purposes. The early Egyptians were one of the first civilizations to use this substance for mummification, cleaning, and personal hygiene. In the early 20th Century it was frequently used to treat colds and the flu, with many reporting remarkable recoveries. It remains one of the cheapest and most versatile substances in any household.

Did You Know? Some of the most common uses of Baking Soda:
– Used in cooking as a leavening agent.
– Widely used as an antacid for indigestion, heartburn and an upset stomach.
– Commonly used in laundry detergents and as an overall disinfectant for cleaning sinks, bathrooms, and other household surfaces.
– Strong antifungal and antiparasitical agent in the colon.
– It helps the kidneys get rid of uric acid, and helps prevent gout and kidney stones.
– Used to treat acidosis in the hospital, amongst other things.
– Commonly used in place of toothpaste for whitening teeth and as an ingredient in some toothpaste brands.

> – May be used to treat bee and bug bites.
> – It is a well-known stain remover on clothing and carpets.
> – It can be used as an exfoliate on the skin.

Even after a century of replacing holistic medical approaches with modern pharmacology, traditional medicine still uses sodium bicarbonate in the hospital. It is employed to treat metabolic acidosis, a very dangerous acidic level in the body, by slowing loss of kidney function and improving patient nutritional status.[1] Hospitals also use sodium bicarbonate to treat various drug overdoses, excessive potassium levels, crush injuries, positional asphyxia and Taser injuries.[2] Sodium bicarbonate is an important medicine used by emergency medical technicians and emergency rooms throughout the world, specifically in heart attack patients. The use of sodium bicarbonate in conjunction with epinephrine is well studied since 1968, and is an extremely effective treatment for out of hospital cardiac arrests when chest compressions and Automated External Defibrillators do not work.[3] Cardiac arrest causes the body to produce excessive amounts of lactic acid resulting in acidosis. Sodium bicarbonate quickly reverses this condition.

So how does sodium bicarbonate neutralize lactic acid? When sodium bicarbonate is taken orally, it interacts with hydrochloric acid in the stomach and produces sodium, carbon dioxide and bicarbonate. The bicarbonate is what is absorbed into the body and its pH is about 8.5.[4] When bicarbonate is introduced into the body to treat a heart attack, it converts the excess lactic acid into a form of carbonic acid, which then breaks down into carbon dioxide (CO_2) and water. Excess CO_2 is absorbed into blood plasma, taken to the lungs and expelled. Excess water is removed by the lymphatic system.[5] The ability of sodium bicarbonate to safely and quickly change the body's pH from a dangerous acidic state into a more neutral state is why it is such a powerful medicine.

Although not recognized as a cancer treatment in Western medicine, one study showed sodium bicarbonate effective in reducing side effects and weight loss when used as a pre-treatment for intravenous Cisplatin in treating animal cancers.[6] In holistic medicine however, sodium bicarbonate is used for treating fungal and parasitic infections of the digestive tract, diabetes, and numerous other diseases, including cancer.

> **Did You Know?** A Hindu medical book, the Astanga Hrdayam, in its

first volume of three, the Sutra Sthana & Sarira Sthana, was written over 1,000 years ago and prescribes "alkali of strong potency" to treat cancer.[7]

Now it's time to take a look at a world-renowned, yet controversial oncologist who claims to have successfully treated numerous cancer patients with sodium bicarbonate.

Doctor Tullio Simoncini

Before we discus Doctor Simoncini, let's review what we previously learned about the metabolism of cancer and its byproduct. Cancer does not require oxygen for cell metabolism but uses the fermentation of glucose. The byproduct is lactic acid, resulting in a highly acidic environment within and around the tumor. Just imagine if sodium bicarbonate is introduced directly into an acidic tumor? It would quickly change the pH of the tumor, inhibit fermentation and cause the tumor to die.

This is precisely the concept used by Doctor Tullio Simoncini, a certified Oncologist in Rome, Italy, to create one of the most earth shattering and controversial cancer treatments of the last one hundred years.

Doctor Simoncini claims to have healed numerous patients, including those with later stage disease, using sodium bicarbonate therapy. He asserts that taking sodium bicarbonate orally can be effective against cancer, but it is much more effective if it is delivered in high doses intravenously, particularly if injected into the vein that leads directly to the tumor.[8]

Depending on the tumor, he typically injects a 5 to 8.4 percent solution of sodium bicarbonate into a catheter, which is threaded into an artery that leads directly to the tumor.[9] This is referred to as Intra Arterial Therapy (IAT). However, the catheter is not required for breast, brain and bladder cancer. For breast cancer a small incision can be used to directly inject sodium bicarbonate into the tumor and the area around the tumor. For bladder cancer the sodium bicarbonate can be delivered using a urethral catheter, which is easier to accomplish than a vein catheter. He believes 99 percent of breast and bladder cancer can be healed using this method with no traditional cancer treatment required. He also claims to have experienced amazing success treating brain cancer patients with sodium bicarbonate injected intravenously.[10] This is a remarkable discovery, especially as a potential treatment for brain cancer, because sodium bicarbonate can cross the blood-brain barrier.[11] Simoncini's sodium bicarbonate therapy is extremely safe if taken orally at low dosages. However, intravenous infusions, and trans-dermal ones, meaning through the skin, must be done carefully under the supervision of a doctor.[12]

Simoncini also proposes a fungus theory of cancer, which is way beyond orthodox oncology. He contends that all tumors present the same pathology as a Candida albicans, meaning white fungus. They are like Candida, according to Simoncini, because they are always strikingly white in color and they branch out from the main tumor in a web like pattern. Like cancer, Candida is also very opportunistic, exploiting weak cellular areas of the body, such as damaged cells in the lungs from smoking. At some point, the fungus learns to evade the body's immune system by sealing itself off from normal tissue and disguising itself. Cancer is just like Candida because it is extremely adaptable in learning how to change at the cellular level to evade antigens. According to Simoncini, this explains why cancerous tumors learn to become resistant to chemotherapy. They are simply behaving as all Candida do. When compared to the conventional notion of cancer, Candida appears to be dramatically similar. Certain types of candida are also extremely drug resistant, just like cancer. It seems to be a strong argument, yet it continues to fall on deaf ears in conventional cancer treatment circles.

> **Note**: The fungus theory of cancer is explained in a separate document on Doctor Simoncini's website: http://www.curenaturalicancro.com/en. If you take the time to read this document, it is very helpful to have a background in chemistry and biology to follow what he is trying to say.

Aside from Doctor Simoncini's fungus theory of cancer, he has clinically treated numerous cancer patients successfully with sodium bicarbonate therapy. He claims that his therapy is effective for almost all cancers except bone cancer and melanoma. He also proposes an alternative therapy for skin cancer, using a unique procedure. He reports excellent results treating skin cancer topically with a 7 percent red iodine tincture solution. The red iodine protocol is outlined clearly on his website.

In an interview, Doctor Simoncini was asked if he had an epiphany at some point in his medical career that caused him to understand that cancer could be treated with sodium bicarbonate. He said, "Yes, I was working in a pediatric oncology clinic and all the children were suffering terribly from the chemo and radiation treatment. I watched them slowly die in pain. So I prayed to God and asked him to give me insight on how to rescue these children from the suffering and to save their lives, and God answered me."[13] Following is the URL with this interview: https://www.youtube.com/watch?v=OnrxN4N5KCk

Unfortunately, Doctor Simoncini's non-conventional approach to treating cancer patients did not receive rave reviews in Italy, so they revoked his license to practice medicine, labeled him a quack, and subjected him to constant legal and public attack. Still, there are numerous testimonies of patients, claiming Doctor Simoncini healed them with sodium bicarbonate.

You can find these testimonies on Doctor Simoncini's website and YouTube. I invite you to take the time to read these testimonies and form your own opinion.

Did You Know?
There is a holistic remedy that has been circulated on the Internet for years that claims that by combining baking soda with maple syrup or molasses it can be used as an effective treatment for cancer. The idea is to trick the tumor into taking in the molasses with the bicarbonate molecule attached to it, thus swallowing a highly alkaline poison pill. The problem with this myth is that the sodium bicarbonate is broken down into sodium, carbon dioxide, and bicarbonate by the hydrochloric acid in the stomach. The maple syrup does not bond with the bicarbonate when it is absorbed into the blood. The receptors on the cancer cells will only take in the glucose molecule, not the bicarbonate. However, raising the pH outside the tumor may in fact inhibit its progression into surrounding tissue.

Although the American Cancer Society, among many other western researchers and oncologists, completely refute Simoncini's fungus theory of cancer, there remains a sliver of hope from Simoncini's broken glass, in so much as not everyone has given up on his unorthodox ideas and treatments. There are a small group of researchers in the United States exploring Simoncini's claims, to see if it stands up to laboratory and clinical testing. If they are successful, it could lead to a major advance in treating cancer.

Sodium Bicarbonate Research

A number of studies performed in the United States by a small group of researchers, suggest that changing the pH environment of the human body by making it slightly more alkaline, might produce a buffer that resists a tumor's ability to invade contiguous tissue. In fact, these experiments strongly suggest that some of Doctor Simoncini's claims are correct.

First, let's look at prior research done in the laboratory with live cancer cells. Not surprisingly, this work leans heavily on Doctor Warburg's findings almost a century ago.

It goes like this: Cancer cells prefer fermentation of glucose for cell metabolism in contrast to normal cells, which exclusively use oxygen. Cancer cells have a much higher metabolic rate than normal cells. The byproduct of this high metabolic rate is excessive production of lactic acid, which makes the cellular environment within the tumor acidic. Lactic acid spills outside the tumor into local tissue and this creates a cellular ecosystem favorable for the tumor to expand deeper into the body.

According to researchers at the Moffitt Cancer Center in Tampa, Florida,

> Because the blood supply in tumors is disorganized, a lot of this acid doesn't make it into the blood right away and diffuses into the surrounding tissue. Thus, tumors are not only acidic they also export acid into surrounding tissue. We believe that this export of acid enables tumor cells to invade into surrounding normal tissues as tumors grow.[14]

If this theory is correct, then changing the pH in the cells outside the tumor should produce a buffer that hinders the tumor from expanding into local tissue and lymph nodes. This is exactly what their laboratory research substantiated.

But something that works in the laboratory does not necessarily translate to living organisms; hence, a second tier of testing is required in animals. If successful, it will lead to studies using humans.

Let's look at another study, this one done using animals. In a collaborative effort, researchers from the Moffitt Cancer Center,

University of Arizona, and Wayne State University, performed a groundbreaking study by taking prior laboratory findings that proved sodium bicarbonate could buffer a tumor from spreading locally and to distant areas, and extended this research to the laboratory using mice. Following is an excerpt of their findings:

> Here, we show that oral NaHCO(3) [sodium bicarbonate] selectively increased the pH of tumors and reduced the formation of spontaneous metastases in mouse models of metastatic breast cancer. This treatment regimen was shown to significantly increase the extracellular pH [reduced acidity], but not the intracellular pH of tumors. . . . [Sodium bicarbonate] therapy also reduced the rate of lymph node involvement, yet did not affect the levels of circulating tumor cells. . . .[15]

They also discovered that when sodium bicarbonate is injected into a vein, it inhibits the formation of metastases in prostate cancer cells but not in melanoma cells.

Their findings on prostate cancer and melanoma exactly reproduce those of Doctor Simoncini, that sodium bicarbonate inhibits metastases in prostate cancer, but not in melanoma.

Did You Know? The FDA requires a rigorous process before approving treatments for cancer. Clinical studies with humans are the pinnacle step in determining if the therapy is safe and effective. Clinical trials must go through multiple phases of research and testing, including release of their findings into scientific journals for peer review.

The time it takes to go from initial laboratory testing to the final phase of human trials takes years and can cost hundreds of millions of dollars. Very few of the so-called promising breakthroughs in cancer get very far unless they receive the full support of the FDA and the cancer industry. Suffice it to say, it would not be excessive to liken the process of bringing a promising new therapy to market to sitting in your yard all day watching the grass grow.

Keep in mind that only synthetically manufactured drugs are allowed to compete in the cancer treatment industry. The truth is, if something effective against cancer comes out of the ground, grows on a tree, or comes from a leaf, it is forever condemned to the outer darkness of the cancer market place. The problem is they can't patent or copyright nature.

Please do not blame the people who treat us for this situation—it is not their fault.

In other research, the University of Arizona Cancer Center is conducting clinical trials using breast cancer patients. They are evaluating the effects of sodium bicarbonate on relieving the pain of patients with bone cancer, and also performing a Phase 1/2 study that will administer sodium bicarbonate orally to patients who are concurrently undergoing chemotherapy using Gemcitabine for metastatic pancreatic cancer.

Like the University of Arizona, Moffitt Cancer Center is advancing this research in an encouraging direction. They are in the midst of groundbreaking clinical research with pancreatic cancer patients using sodium bicarbonate as a buffer to determine if the same effects in animals are present in humans.[16] Pancreatic cancer comes with the worst possible prognosis and any progress made in treating this very dangerous cancer would be extraordinary. Researchers at Moffitt reference Doctor Simoncini's work, but dispel his theory on cancer being a fungus; yet, they do make a point of saying that his observational findings "do not make him or his ideas wrong."[17]

The Soaking Protocol

The esophagus is an organ with an internal membrane made up of epithelial cells, which are a type of skin cell. The skin on our body has multiple layers. The outermost layer consists of very dense dead-skin cells, which provide a waterproof barrier. If this were not the case we would dry up like a prune very quickly and die.

Nevertheless, the skin is still a membrane and fat-soluble substances, like some oils, can be absorbed into the skin and cause an allergic reaction or even poison us. Good examples of this are Poison Ivy and fossil fuel based solvents. In contrast, the epithelial cells of the esophagus do not have a tough outer layer and are much more permeable. Scattered under the epithelial layer of the esophagus are submucosal glands. These glands work throughout the day pumping mucous over the esophagus to protect it from gastric acid and acidic food.[18,19] When the esophagus is exposed to too much acid on a regular basis, the protection breaks down and the cells get damaged. Take a guess as to what protective substance is in the mucous? It is bicarbonate!

Knowing this made it an easy leap for me to try soaking the epithelial layers of the esophagus with sodium bicarbonate in an attempt to alkalize the esophagus and promote healing. During radiation therapy I was able to eat solid foods for the entire course of treatment, which surprised all of my doctors.

The protocol I developed was to mix one half to one teaspoon of Baking Soda with four ounces of water and lie on my back and swallow one small sip at a time to let it slowly work its way over the affected areas. I always did this on an empty stomach because taking baking soda on a full stomach can be dangerous. I would rotate my body about 1/8 of a turn, take a sip, and do it again until I rotated my body 360 degrees. I did this protocol two to three times a day, from five weeks prior to treatment, all the way through treatment, and for about six weeks post-treatment. Treating my esophagus in this manner also allowed me to easily keep my body pH between 7.5 and 8.0, using very little additional baking soda.

Let's now look at the cautions Arm & Hammer publishes on their Baking Soda box.

Arm & Hammer Baking Soda Box
- Ask a doctor before use if you have a sodium-restricted diet.
- Ask a doctor or pharmacist before use if you are taking a prescription drug or antacid.
- Do not administer to children under the age of five.
- To avoid serious injury, do not take until powder is dissolved.
- It is dangerous to take this product if overly full from food or drink.
- Consult a doctor if severe stomach pain occurs taking this product.
- Stop use and ask a doctor if symptoms last more than two weeks.
- Directions: add ½ teaspoon to 4 ounces of water and take every 2 hours, or as directed by a physician.
- Do not take more than 7 doses, or 3 and ½ tsps in a 24-hour period.
- If over 60 years old, do not take more that 3 and ½ doses or 2 teaspoons in a 24 hour period.
- Do not take the maximum dose for more than 2 weeks.

Doctor Mark Sircus, an expert on the use of sodium bicarbonate as medicine for treating all sorts of illnesses, reinforces Doctor Simoncini's ideas. Doctor Sircus states that one week of elevated pH should be followed by one week off to let your pH stabilize back to normal, and that one should not let the pH exceed 8.0 for any prolonged periods because it can cause serious health issues, including serious harm to the kidney and bladder. He states that the key to safely monitoring pH is through testing urine and saliva several times a day using pH strips.[20]

Although sodium bicarbonate therapy is safe if performed following Arm and Hammers' cautions, there are other things we should be aware of, according to Doctor Sircus.

Other Precautions

Raising the body's pH too high for too long can cause alkalosis, a potentially life threatening situation.[21] Doctor Sircus sites key symptoms of alkalosis as confusion, light-headedness, numbness or tingling in the face or extremities, nausea, vomiting, hand tremor, muscle twitching, or prolonged muscle spasms.[22] When I first experimented with sodium bicarbonate I intentionally got my pH well over 8.0 for about three days in a row and experienced some light headedness and tingling in my face. The first symptom I usually experienced, when I was taking too much sodium bicarbonate, was diarrhea. It cleared up as soon as I stopped taking the bicarbonate.

Too high a pH can cause hypernatremia, a dangerously high sodium level in the blood.[23] Individuals with chronic pulmonary problems, kidney problems, severe edema, liver or kidney disease, and high blood pressure should avoid it.[24] It should be done the first thing in the morning on an empty stomach and right before bed each night, within three hours after eating. If done during the day, it should be done between meals.[25] Taking sodium bicarbonate on a full stomach can cause the stomach to rupture and put one in a life or death situation.[26] If there is any doubt about allergies, or any other health problem, a physician should be consulted first.

Although there are a lot of precautions with using sodium bicarbonate, it remains a safe natural substance for most people if used carefully, and this includes the need for buying pH strips and testing urine several times a day. I stopped testing saliva because it does not change much during the day and the pH level in the urine changes throughout the day. A normal urine pH in the morning is slightly acidic, between 6.0 and 7.0 and it should become more alkaline as the day progresses, reaching 7.5 to 8.0 by the evening, according to Doctor Sircus.

Most people have very acidic diets and measure 6.0 and below in the morning. This requires them to take higher doses of bicarbonate. It was not difficult to get my pH over 7.5 every day from just being on an alkaline diet. In fact, it was easy to push it over 8.0 with a little baking soda. Do not be surprised to see a pH level between 4.0 and 5.0 if you have cancer, or are in treatment for cancer, because cancer coupled with chemo and radiation makes the body very acidic.

Kits for testing pH are available on the Internet. They come in packs of 100. Testing urine is the most accurate when the pH strip is dipped into a sample of urine in a small plastic cup. Putting the strip into a stream will cause the colors to bleed over, resulting in a false reading.

Finally, Doctor Simoncini contends that any tumor that is exposed in the mouth, throat, esophagus, stomach or digestive tract is a candidate for oral sodium bicarbonate therapy, and if done carefully, is safe. There are no doctors practicing this therapy in the United States because it is not an FDA approved cancer therapy.

For those interested in Intra Arterial Therapy (IAT) the Europa Institute, in Tijuana, Mexico, offers cesium chloride IAT, which is an alkaline substance with even higher alkalinity than sodium bicarbonate. This institute also offers a whole array of other alternative and holistic cancer therapies.

Summary

Doctor Simoncini is a remarkable man. His success in treating cancer patients with sodium bicarbonate is well established. Yet, his cancer treatment protocols and fungus theory remain controversial. The American Cancer Society, among many other Western researchers and oncologists, entirely refute his fungus theory of cancer and for the most part dismiss sodium bicarbonate as a possible treatment for cancer. To be honest, I only care about the practicality of whether sodium bicarbonate can be an effective chemical agent against Barrett's Esophagus and cancer. My personal experience is that I believe it played a key role in resolving my Barrett's Esophagus and perhaps in helping contain my tumor while I awaited treatment. The fact that cancer produces an acidic ecosystem within and outside a tumor is substantial enough to deserve serious attention. As far as the fungus theory of cancer goes, let's leave it to the biochemists and move on.

Revolutionary clinical research is currently underway in the United States to determine if sodium bicarbonate, or other alkali substances can be used as a buffer against cancer invading local tissue, the lymphatic system and to distant metastasis. If this current work proves correct, the implications are enormous. It would be a major breakthrough in understanding how cancer spreads and it might also offer a more effective therapy to prolong life and cure cancer. Yet, sodium bicarbonate therapy remains far from FDA approval.

I remain hopeful that current research will lead to a breakthrough in treating cancer. I offer my personal testimony as one additional data point that invites researchers to initiate further study on whether sodium bicarbonate soakings can actually reverse Barrett's Esophagus, and also act as a buffer against tumors. Even more so, imagine how safe it might be to perform a number of clinical studies that inject sodium bicarbonate transdermally into the tumors of breast cancer patients, and also endoscopic injection of sodium bicarbonate into mouth, throat, esophageal and gastric tumors.

Perhaps one day, the money gods in Washington, D.C., who control the cancer research purse strings and the approval process for novel cancer therapies, will take note of the work done by Doctor Simoncini and others and connect it to what Albert Einstein once luminously quipped, "When the solution is simple, God is answering."

Notes

1. Bankhead, Charles. "Bicarbonate Slows Chronic Kidney Disease," NEPHROLOGY 07.16.2009, http://www.medpagetoday.com/Nephrology/ESRD/15113 (accessed December 30, 2015, 1).
2. Davis, Jim, MA, RN, EMT-P, "Sodium Bicarbonate, Should It Be Considered As A Treatment?," Nov 30, 2010, The Journal of Emergency Medical Services, http://www.jems.com/articles/print/volume-35/issue-12/patient-care/sodium-bicarbonate.html (accessed December 30, 2015, 8).
3. Ibid., 6-7.
4. Sircus, Mark. Using The Healing Power OF Baking Soda: Sodium Bicarbonate, Nature's Unique First Aid Remedy. Garden City Park, New York: Square One Publishers, 2014, 106.
5. Ibid., 2.
6. Guindon J et al. "Optimization of a cisplatin model of chemotherapy-induced peripheral neuropathy in mice: use of vitamin C and sodium bicarbonate pretreatments to reduce nephrotoxicity and improve animal health status," Abstract, Mol Pain, 2014 Sep 4;10:56. doi: 10.1186/1744-8069-10-56, http://www.ncbi.nlm.nih.gov/pubmed/25189223 (accessed December 30, 2015).
7. "Treating Cancer & Destroying Tumors With Baking Soda," Healing Cancer Naturally, August 2007, http://www.healingcancernaturally.com/sodium-bicarbonate-treatment.html (accessed January 8, 2016).
8. "Sodium Bicarbonate Treatment," http://www.curenaturalicancro.com/en/sodium-bicarbonate-treatment (accessed December 18, 2015).
9. Ibid.
10. Doug Kaufman Interview of Doctor Tullio Simoncini, "Cancer is a Fungus 2 of 2," https://www.youtube.com/watch?v=OnrxN4N5KCk (accessed December 30, 2015).
11. Davis, 6.
12. Deeken JF, Loscher, W. "The blood-brain barrier and cancer: transporters, treatment, and Trojan horses," Abstract, Clinical Cancer Res. 2007 Mar 15;13(6):1663-74, http://www.ncbi.nlm.nih.gov/pubmed/17363519 (accessed December 30, 2015).
13. Ibid.
14. "Buffer Therapy," Research Projects. Moffitt Cancer Center,

Department of Imagining and Metabolism, http://imaging.moffitt.org/research-4.aspx (accessed January 7, 2016, 1).

15. Robey, IF et al. "Bicarbonate Increases Tumor pH and Inhibits Spontaneous Metastases," Cancer Res. 2009 Mar 15;69(6):2260-8. doi: 10.1158/0008-5472.CAN-07-5575. Epub 2009 Mar 10. Abstract, http://www.ncbi.nlm.nih.gov/pubmed/19276390 (accessed December 18, 2015).

16. Gatenby, Rovert A., Gillies, Robert J. "Research Projects: Buffer Therapy," Moffitt Cancer Center, Department of Cancer Imaging and Metabolism, http://imaging.moffitt.org/research-4.aspx (accessed December 30, 2015, 1-2.).

17. Ibid., 2.

18. Long, John D., Orlando, Roy C., "Esophageal Submucosal Glands: Structure and Function," American Journal of Gastroenterology 94, 2818 -2824 (October 1999) | doi:10.1111/j.1572-0241.1999.1422_b.x, 1-2.

19. Weisenberg, Elliot, M.D., "Esophagus General Histology," 2003-2013, PathologyOutlines.com, Inc. http://www.pathologyoutlines.com/topic/esophagusnormalhistology.html (accessed January 9, 2016, 1).

20. Ibid., 155.

21. Sircus, 144.

22. Ibid., 158.

23. Ibid., 156.

24. Ibid., 157, 159.

25. Ibid., 156.

26. Ibid.

CHAPTER 13

The Moment of Truth

*The Lord's loving kindness never ceases, His mercies
never come to an end, they are new every morning . . . .*
—Lamentations 3:22-24

March 7, 2014 came quickly. It was Wednesday afternoon, almost six weeks following chemo-radiation when I met with my surgeon, Doctor S. for the third time. This meeting entailed a final assessment in preparation for the esophagectomy, scheduled two days later. The morning consisted of blood work and a CT-PET scan, and both were clean. I vacillated as to whether to call the surgery off or proceed with it, right up to the moment I walked into his office that day. Stepping off the elevator with Kelly it occurred to me, "These guys are going to get really ticked off if I pull myself off the surgery schedule." We had developed a strong connection with Doctor S., and the thought of disappointing him made the weight on my shoulders even heavier.

Doctor S. walked into our room, sat down and immediately congratulated me on a clean PET scan. Then he said, "Looks like you are in good shape to do the surgery this Friday. Are you ready to go?" I adjusted my glasses and responded, "I'm not sure if I'm ready to go through with the surgery, and would really like to first have an upper endoscopy and to take some biopsies and see how well my esophagus healed. If things don't look good I will do the surgery, but if everything is healed up, then I want to opt out of the surgery." As Doctor S. stood up, his jaw dropped. He then walked closer to me, crossed his arms, looked me in the eyes, and said, "I want you to feel good about the surgery, but I think you are making a mistake if you opt out of it. I have never seen an undamaged esophagus following radiation and chemotherapy and there is too much risk that the cancer might come back if we don't take it out." I replied, "I realize that, but I believe there is a good chance my esophagus healed from all of the holistic things I've been doing." He paused, and then said, "O.K., I'll tell you what we can do. I'll refer you to Doctor G., a Gastroenterologist who works closely with us. He has worked with esophageal cancer patients for years and can give you a second opinion, examine your esophagus and then you can decide. How does that sound?" I said, "That sounds great, let's do it." He quickly replied, "But if Doctor G. finds anything questionable, then you will go ahead with the surgery . . . right?" "Yes," I said, "it's a deal." On our walk back to the car Kelly commented, "Joe, I think you're doing the right thing, and besides, if it comes back you can always do the surgery, unless it's metastatic." "You're right," I said, "and that's a risk I'm willing to take right now."

When I met with my oncologist the following day he said, "We have never seen anyone opt out of the surgery after being medically cleared for it. You are a rare case." Doctor O. remained as insistent as Doctor S. that I go ahead with the surgery for fear of a metastatic recurrence. I explained to him a recent study that I had read, stating that surgery following chemo-radiation is controversial,[1] especially for early stage cancers, and that the rate of recurrence in the long-term was not much different between the two options. He responded, "Joe, the surgery is a critical element, but I think a second opinion and the endoscopy are good things that will give you peace of mind." Later that same day I met with my Radiologist, who gave me the same exhortation to do the surgery.

The following week I met with the Gastroenterologist, Doctor G., and just like my other three doctors, he gave an impassioned argument as to why I should not opt out of the surgery. He based it upon a number of esophageal cancer patients of his, who had chemo and radiation but were not medically able to have the surgery. They subsequently experienced a metastatic recurrence and died within months. I listened to Doctor G. and almost gave in, but Kelly said, "Joe, having the endoscopy will give you peace of mind." On that perspicuous note, Doctor G. honored my desire, and within a week I was back under the thrall of Propofol.

The night before the endoscopy I tossed and turned all night in bed. Clouded with uncertainty, my mind raced back and forth over the consequences of making the wrong decision. The words of Doctor G. haunted me, "My most recent patient died within three months of recurrence." So did the words of Doctor R., "Radiation damage to the esophagus is irreversible." At least three nurses had also questioned my judgment asking, "How badly do you want to live." Yet, the people closest to me, my wife, mom and dad, kids, brothers and some close friends urged me to avoid the surgery. They all said the same thing, that they had a bad feeling about the surgery for me. They all believed I would be healed. I pondered all these things and rolled out of bed that morning exhausted and emotionally drained.

After showering, I shuffled towards the aroma of freshly brewed hazelnut-flavored coffee. The smell paired nicely with my body's desire to shake off the sleepless night. The procedure was scheduled for 1:00 pm that afternoon. I had about five hours to get my head right. Kelly swiveled out of the laundry room into the kitchen and immediately saw the angst on my face and asked, "How are you doing this morning, is everything O.K.?" I said, "I had a rough night last night and didn't sleep at all. "I've been praying for days for an answer and haven't received a thing. All I hear is silence. I've changed my mind and think it would be foolish for me to go against the advice of my doctors. They don't have a cure for recurrent cancer if it's metastatic. I have no other option because I don't know enough about alternative cancer therapies to even think of trying one of those." She looked at me contemplatively and said, "Are you really sure about this? Why don't you wait until you see the results of the endoscopy? At least you'll have peace of mind that the surgery is justified." I replied, I keep asking God to give me an answer, to show me a sign, any sign, and all I hear is silence." She said, "Joe, please be patient and give this a little more time." I said, "O.K., but I'm going to need a huge fleece from Doctor G. He will have to literally tell me that I have a brand new esophagus. Anything short of that and I feel as though I have to go through with the surgery." She said, "Joe, I feel real good about this, so let's just trust God with it, and besides, we will get our answer this afternoon." I was wrong about God being silent in regard to giving guidance on what I should do. He was speaking to me through Kelly and I wasn't listening.

By 2:30 that afternoon, I was in the recovery room waking up. I remember lying there and not seeing any nurses or Kelly nearby. I was alone. I remember thinking, "The moment of truth has arrived." Seconds later Doctor G. emerged out of a hallway and shuffled towards me. As he approached my bed, he took off his glasses, grinned from ear to ear and said, "Mister Marx, it looks like you have a brand new esophagus." I was stunned. I didn't know what to say, except, "Thank you." He just repeated the exact same words I gave Kelly earlier that morning for the fleece I needed from God. He said, "You did really well with the procedure and I have never seen anything like this. Your esophagus did not have any scar tissue from the site of the tumor, nor was there any damage to the surrounding tissue. I want to debrief you and Kelly in about an hour, following my last procedure of the day. I told the nurse to get the discharge paperwork done and take you to the meeting room next to the lobby." I said, "Thank you Doctor G. for the wonderful news."

Kelly and I were amazed at Doctor G.'s testimony during the debriefing. He said, "Joe, I have never seen anything like this in over 17 years of practicing medicine. Your esophagus looks like it could be either Kelly's or mine. It looks brand new. You have a little inflammation down there but there is no scar tissue, no sign of radiation damage, nor is there any evidence that there was ever a tumor in that location. I also did not see any Barrett's Esophagus, which is astonishing. I took multiple biopsies of the lower esophagus and will get back to you with the results in a couple of days, but I would be surprised to see any cancerous or pre-cancerous tissue in the report." I profusely thanked him for taking such good care of us. He said, "I am going to call Doctor S. later today and give this report to him personally. If the pathology report is negative, I will support your wish to opt out of the surgery, and instead, go under very close surveillance over the next year." So the moment of truth had arrived—and mercy found us.

Notes

1. "Radiation Therapy and Esophageal Cancer", Ravi Shridhar, MD, et al, Journal of the Moffett Cancer Center, Cancer Control.2013;20 (2):97-110, p. 12, http://Medscape.com/viewarticle/782537_12 (accessed November 11, 2015).

CHAPTER 14

Preventing Recurrence

The best cure for one's bad tendencies is to see
them in action in another person.
—Alain de Botton

Getting cancer is sort of like experiencing a head on collision with a truck. It may not kill you instantly but it will sure enough try to kill you. With cancer however, you face an additional threat. As the old saying goes, "If the cancer doesn't kill you, the treatment will." Getting through cancer treatment is only the beginning of a lifelong endeavor to escape its clutches. If we embrace our unfortunate situation head on, with a smile on our face, and realize there are holistic things that we can do to prevent recurrence and heal from the side effects, then hope will arise. Are you ready to learn how to take control of your cancer in the post treatment period? Let's get started.

To begin, what is the difference between a recurring cancer and a secondary one? A recurring cancer means that cells from the original tumor become active again, and this happens more often than not in the early months or years following treatment. A recurring cancer can occur in the local area of the original tumor or it may spread to some other area of the body. In comparison, a secondary cancer means a different species of cancer sprouts in an area local to the original tumor, or in an area removed from it.

What specifically should be done to prevent recurrence? In general, the answer is simple, and that is to maintain a healthy body ecology. The first part of this chapter will review the holistic practices we previously learned with an emphasis on how important they are for the rest of our lives to prevent recurrence. This requires a commitment to maintain good eating and lifestyle habits. In spite of this, it is not such an easy thing to do. The mind can be easily tricked by the flesh, into believing something that is bad for the body is not so bad. This is where we all get into trouble. When we look in the mirror we need to have the conviction to call a strike when we see a strike, and a ball when we see a ball. If we don't, our bad habit-dancing partner might waltz us right into the hospital or grave.

In addition to maintaining good diet and lifestyle habits, we need to understand the nature of any treatment-induced side effects we experience and develop a game plan to cure them. Why? Side effects weaken our body and make us more susceptible to recurrence. However, they present a tricky variable in the healing algorithm. They are one of the most difficult areas to manage, to the extent traditional medicine does not address them except when they are very serious or life threatening. Consequently, the threat of a treatment-induced cancer is very real but few patients understand this threat.

Ignoring side effects by simply learning to live with them, or because no one else seems concerned, is not a winning approach. The second part of this chapter addresses how to deal with treatment-provoked injuries, euphemistically referred to as side effects, to help prevent recurrence and secondary cancers. It also proposes various research-based holistic approaches to mitigate, and potentially heal, a number of the more common side effects.

Developing an informed treatment plan that addresses all of one's side effects is not something that can be done detached from the counsel of an expert. For those who seek to do everything in their power to live, consultation with a health specialist in naturopathic or alternative cancer treatment is profitable. Consulting with a non-conventional doctor is also an opportunity to better understand the scope of alternative therapies that might be available should conventional treatment fail. The third part of this chapter speaks to the benefit of seeking consultation with a secondary tier of experts to assist in managing the side effects.

Again, if we choose to ignore the side effects and simply try to coexist with them, or we go back to harmful diet and lifestyle habits, or we go back to a stressful job or life situation, then for all intents and purposes, we will be contributing to a body ecology that invites cancer to come back.

Habits That Help Prevent Recurrence

In post treatment surveillance, one's mettle is tested as to whether they revert back to cancer promoting eating and lifestyle habits. This is particularly true for those who experience a complete therapeutic response and the cancer is in remission, since this can lull us into a false sense of security. The farther one gets from the completion of treatment, the easier it is to sow the seeds of complacency. Complacency is a strange bedfellow with holistic health habits, so there remains no other choice than to be vigilant.

Let's review the researched based, holistic approaches to diet and lifestyle that can resist cancer, those things discussed earlier in this book, including a few things elaborated on in the next chapter. This list is only a framework for each patient to build his or her own personalized post treatment plan.

1. Balanced Alkaline Diet, Incorporating:
   – No Sugar or Refined Starches
   – No Dairy (casein promotes cancer growth)
   – Purge Inflammatory Foods
   – Fresh Fruit and Vegetables (no processed foods)
   – Low Animal Protein
   – Low to Moderate Good Oils (such as olive and flaxseed oil)
   – Diet Rich in Cruciferous Vegetables (promotes glutathione production, the most important antioxidant that resists cancer)
   – Periodic Fasting (weekly or monthly), or Intermittent Fasting (eating all meals between a four to six hour window each day, see Chapter 14)
2. Healthy Life Style Choices (no tobacco or substance abuse)
3. Daily Exercise (30 minutes of aerobic exercise, 5 days a week, even if it is only daily walks)
4. Targeted Natural Substances: Especially effective using the Greece Tests, in particular, the Onconomics Plus (see Chapter 14).

5. Detoxification and Probiotics

6. Filtered Water

7. Plenty of Rest

8. Low Stress Job

9. Spirituality

10. Detoxify the home and workspace from radio frequency and electro magnetic smog, and certain cancer causing substances in home interior products, children's toys, cleaning substances, cosmetics and hygiene products. Check the labels on all home and personal use products for warning signs on toxicity and guaranties of product safety on human health.

For instance, the Stetzerizer electro-magnetic forces (EMF) filter can be plugged into any 120V outlet and it will clean dirty electricity and substantially reduce exposure to excessive EMF. A meter is purchased with the filters to survey the current fields at each receptacle throughout the house. A safe level is below 25 and I had readings of over 400 in my house. After installing these filters my daughter said her migraine headaches greatly diminished and I started sleeping more soundly. A number of companies sell these on the Internet.

Managing Chemo and Radiation Induced Injuries

As difficult as it is at times to accept a well known, but unpleasant fact about something that seriously affects our health, it is more difficult o force our self to do something about it. Most cancer patients are aware of the fact that chemotherapeutic drugs and radiation therapy damage the DNA of millions of normal cells; yet they too easily remove themselves from the reality that some of these cells may one day turn cancerous. In part, the cancer treatment system unintentionally downplays the seriousness of the side effects to help us get through treatment. If they told us every single detail about how awful the side effects might be, many of us might not go through with the treatment. This conditions us to believe that the treatment isn't so bad—don't sweat the small potatoes. It gives the patient an out. If the only side effects we need to worry about are the ones that hospitalize us or exclude us from further treatment, then what do we have to worry about, right? It is kind of like that when a doting mother constantly tells her struggling student that the teacher gives too much homework and the teacher is the problem. The consequence of the mother's action is that the student ends up being conditioned to believe that their effort is good enough, and is inadvertently encouraged not to do their homework. The end result is kind of like a side effect, and the student struggles even more. How can we break free from this effect? Understanding how damaging chemo and radiation is on the body and how this damage creates an environment conducive for cancer to return, is a good start.

Side Effects: In General

Most chemotherapeutic drugs are designed to attack cells that reproduce at a high rate. This not only includes cancer cells, it includes cells in our nerves, skin, hair, fingernails, bone marrow, and lining of the mouth, esophagus, and stomach. The result is acute poisoning of healthy cells throughout the body. All chemo drugs are toxic to organs to some extent too, especially the liver, kidneys, bladder, heart, lungs, reproductive system and the brain.[1] The liver is one of the more common organs that is damaged by chemo because the liver acts as a filter and metabolizes the chemicals in the drugs.

Let's look at some of the most common side effects of chemo: hair loss, nausea, vomiting, low blood cell counts, extreme fatigue, decreased mental acuity, constipation, stomach pain, jaw pain, and neuropathy, which is damage to the nerve endings in the extremities, and chemo induced cancer. These side effects will vary depending on the types of drugs the patient is exposed too, and on how well the patient's body can handle them.

One of the most common but least talked about side effects is decreased mental acuity, which includes, clumsiness, loss of memory, poor balance, hearing loss, shaking, difficulty walking, and poor hand to eye coordination.[2]

Likewise, radiation therapy can cause a number of side effects that are similar to chemotherapy, including injury to organs and soft tissue. Radiation therapy is particularly prone to producing secondary cancers at high doses. It is especially dangerous to organs such as the lungs and heart.

Even though I handled chemo-radiation well, my body was damaged in a lot more ways than I had imagined. I suspect this is true for most cancer patients.

Side Effects: My Experience

While the list of side effects covered is by no means comprehensive it should serve as a departure point to help evaluate your own situation. Following are the treatment-induced side effects that I experienced with the holistic approaches I used to help mitigate, and in some cases, heal their effect.

Chemo Fog: One of the most misunderstood, yet widely experienced and debilitating side effects of chemotherapy is reduced cognitive ability. Many in the chemo culture strenuously argue that post treatment cognitive impairment is not related to the toxic drugs that are used. Their explanation is that something else is causing it, but they do not know what that something else is. Look at different sources before you form an opinion, because some of the large organizations that publish these studies either come from, or receive funding from, one of the large pharmaceutical companies, and they seem a little defensive about the possibility of chemo fog being the result of chemo drugs passing through the blood-brain barrier. Those who experience chemo fog will tell you otherwise. It's a no brainer for them.

At any rate, chemo fog or chemo brain, whatever you choose to call it, is not something widely discussed with the patient as a side effect to worry about. It is not considered life threatening—and so, there you have it. In cancer circles it is referred to in a very light-hearted manner. When you are not able to think clearly, or you can't find your car keys, or speak in a complete sentence with subject and predicate, all you have to do is tell your family and friends, "I'm experiencing a little chemo fog. Ha-ha-ha, isn't that funny, my brain doesn't work right anymore?"

By the last week of treatment, my chemo fog was so severe that Kelly would not let me drive a car for the next three to four months. I was petrified by the thought of having to live with some level of permanent cognitive brain damage for the rest of my life. For some however, many of the symptoms from chemo fog will heal within a year or two following treatment. But for others, the side effects can last for years. According to the American Cancer Society,

> The sometimes-vague yet distressing mental changes, cancer patients notice are real, not imagined. They might last a short time, or they might go on for years. These changes can make

people unable to go back to their school, work, or social activities, or make it so that it takes a lot of mental effort to do so. Chemo brain affects everyday life for many people with cancer.[3]

Chemo fog was not really discussed with me prior to treatment and only referred to in a light-hearted manner a few times during treatment. They don't have a cure for it, so I suppose there is not much to say about it other than to try and downplay how bad it might be.

One of the drugs I was treated with was Carboplatin, which is a platinum based drug. It shows up on the Periodic Table as a metal. From my recollection of chemistry, concentrations of platinum, or any other heavy metal in the body can be harmful. Knowing this doesn't necessarily mean my brain was damaged by a platinum-based drug. It could have been from a chemical interaction with the other chemo drug I had—but it makes one highly suspicious.

In a marquee study done by Dartmouth University, scientists discovered that standard dose chemotherapy could impair cognitive ability for up to 10 years after treatment. In this study 128-breast cancer and lymphoma survivors, who had received chemotherapy, were compared to those treated with only surgery or radiation. The patients were all disease free. The chemo group scored significantly lower across multiple domains, especially in the areas of memory, concentration, and ability to integrate different types of information.[4]

I did not handle the reality of this side effect very well. I even fell into a period of despair, wondering if I would ever be able to stand in front of a classroom again and teach. I recall thinking, "I'm not going to let these chemicals disable me. I'm going to exercise and eat my way out of this mess." I knew the value of exercise and a balanced alkaline diet and how they can powerfully purge toxins out of the body and stimulate the production of new cells. Furthermore, there are a number of herbal supplements that are purported to improve brain function, Ginko Biloba and CoQ10 being two of them. There are also certain super foods that have a good reputation in helping cognitive ability, namely, turmeric, wild Alaskan salmon, walnuts, cruciferous vegetables, coconut oil and blueberries.[5] Most of these foods graced my diet in the period following treatment. Fortunately, my chemo fog cleared up substantially within the first year of treatment, but some symptoms persist almost three years later. I took Ginko and CoQ10 at different periods of time, and believe I experienced the most positive impact from CoQ10; but everyone is different, and what works for one person may not work for another.

I also lost my ability to dream, something I had since I was a child. However, after doing several treatments of low dose Pulsed Electro-Magnetic Force (PEMF) therapy to increase blood flow and stimulate white blood cell activity, I experienced an amazing and unexpected result. I started to dream again. In some mysterious way the PEMF helped my brain heal enough to have dreams again.

Neuropathy: One of the most prevalent and potentially long-lasting side effects is peripheral neuropathy, which is loss of feeling from damaged nerve endings in our hands and feet. Almost every chemo patient I have spoken with claims they experienced some level of neuropathy. I experienced about a 90 percent loss of feeling in three fingers and part of the palm of my left hand. It was extremely exasperating trying to type with my left hand on a keyboard. It gave fat-fingering a whole new connotation. To be honest, I wanted to give chemotherapy a Ctl-Alt-Del. Although there are a number of drugs available for diabetic neuropathy, my Oncologist told me that they are not very effective with chemo-induced neuropathy. Amazingly however, something else came to the rescue—PEMF. After a hand full of PEMF treatments, no pun intended, to stimulate my immune system, the neuropathy in my fingers and left hand healed. I still have a little numbness at the tip of my pinky but I have no problem typing again.

Macrocytosis: Macrocytosis is a blood disorder in which red blood cells become enlarged. Although there are many possible causes of Macrocytosis, it is commonly associated with bone marrow or liver damage from chemotherapy. Macrocytosis is a well-known trigger for pre-leukemia or Myelodysplastic Syndrome (MSL). MSL is a manage-able disease in most cases. Yet, up to 33 percent of those who get it will progress to Acute Myelogenous Leukemia (AML), which is not only the most common of the four types of adult leukemia but also the most deadly. One source stated that those who undergo chemotherapy are at risk of getting AML for up to 10 years after treatment. I managed this side effect using diet and exercise and recently added Iron, Folic Acid and B-12 supplements, and a Chinese herbal supplement called Tang-

Kuei Four Combination, produced by Sun Ten Laboratories. After four months the Macrocytosis improved to borderline normal.

Acute Hemolytic Anemia (AHA): AHA is a blood disorder where red blood cells are destroyed at a faster rate than they can be produced. It is a well-known side effect of chemotherapy and is indicative of possible bone marrow damage. This side effect was managed using the same supplements I used for the Macrocytosis. After six weeks on the aforementioned supplements, my Hemoglobin moved up to the low normal value.

Stranding in Lower Lobes of Lungs: Stranding is radiation induced inflammation and scarring of the lungs. I experienced stranding in both of my lower lungs. For breast, esophageal and lung cancer, the lungs are one of the most common places for recurrence. A number of other radiation induced lung injuries can occur, such as pneumonitis, pericarditis, effusions and fibrosis. I also took a supplement recommended by one of my naturopathic doctors called Pneuma-Zyme. The stranding in my lungs has since healed.

Did You Know? The Power of Cruciferous Vegetables

A number of researchers discovered that various nutrients in the cruciferous family of vegetables, which include cauliflower, broccoli, kale, brussel sprouts, and cabbage play a significant role in preventing and slowing the progression of cancer. One of the main anticancer agents in cruciferous vegetables is phytochemicals. One study concluded, "Among the various vegetables, broccoli and other cruciferous species appear most closely associated with reduced cancer risk in organs such as the colorectum, lung, prostate and breast."[6] Other agents in these vegetables, namely, indoles and isothiocyanates, have been found to inhibit the development of cancer in several organs in rats and mice, including the bladder, breast, colon, liver, lung, and stomach."[7] One large Chinese study of breast cancer survivors found a 22 percent improved survival rate for those who consumed the highest amounts of cruciferous vegetables.[8] In a similar study researchers discovered a moderately reduced risk of lung cancer in non-smokers who consumed one serving of cauliflower per day.[9] Recall that cruciferous vegetables provide a strong precursor base for the production of glutathione, the most powerful antioxidant.

Extreme Fatigue: Extreme fatigue is one of the most prevalent side effects of cancer treatment and one of the most difficult to treat. The best remedies for fatigue are a balanced alkaline diet, daily exercise, plenty of sleep, a low stress job, and hydration, because all of these things will help the body heal faster than anything else. Another source of help is to have blood tests done by your primary care doctor, oncologist or some other specialist.

I had my blood extensively tested by both a naturopathic doctor and a degenerative disease specialist. They were able to identify some mineral, vitamin and hormonal deficiencies and put me on some targeted natural supplements and vitamins to help my body deal with fatigue.

Coronary Artery Disease: I experienced calcification in one of my heart valves two years post treatment. This side effect is consistent with a possible radiation therapy induced injury. According to my Cardiologist, when the heart is damaged by radiation, it produces excessive amounts of calcium at the site of the injury to help it heal, which can result in a build up of plaque. With this side effect it is more critical to maintain a plant-based diet and keep cholesterol in a normal range.

High Cholesterol: Following treatment my cholesterol shot up to almost 300, despite the fact I maintained a highly plant-based diet. High cholesterol is frequently the result of a damaged liver. My Radiation Oncologist previously said, "You could lose up to one third of your liver function from radiation therapy." It took almost a year of trying everything except synthetic anti-cholesterol drugs to find a holistic answer for this problem.

To my good fortune, I stumbled across Phyto-Sitosterols, which are a safe, plant-based substance that reportedly improves cholesterol. After taking two grams of Phyto-Sitosterols per day for three months, my LDL dropped from 187 to 115, and my HDL increased to 90. A miracle! Please do not let anyone fool you. There is healing power in nature—complements of the Divine Chemist.

If you are experiencing side effects and have done nothing to help your situation, then by all means educate yourself on this topic and get some professional assistance.

Immune System Suppression: Probably the most ominous side effect of chemo and radiation is significant damage to the body's immune system. If the body is not able to clean up any remaining cancer cells, then the risk of recurrence is extremely high. Equally bad is the risk of secondary cancers, caused by mutation of healthy cells into precancerous cells. Mutated cells can eventually evolve into a treatment-induced cancer.

Chemo, in particular, causes serious and potentially permanent damage to the body's bone marrow—not only its ability to produce both red and white blood cells but also its ability to identify and destroy remaining tumor cells or stem cells. This is one of the primary factors as to why a cancer in remission comes back metastatically. It's also why alternative cancer treatment centers place a high premium on rebuilding the patient's immune system. It also explains why Immunotherapy vaccines offer great promise in treating cancer. They instigate the body's immune system to do something it was no longer capable of doing.

Consult with Naturopathic or Alternative Doctors

One may well ask, what the difference is between Naturopathic and Alternative medicine? Here's the answer. Naturopathic medicine is a form of non-conventional medicine that uses scientifically based approaches for healing. The doctors are trained in conventional medicine but have expertise in naturopathy. Naturopathic medicine does not depend upon surgery or synthetic drugs, and it is frequently referred to as complementary or integrative medicine, because it can easily complement, or be integrated into conventional medicine. It also seeks to treat the whole person in a natural and sensible manner. Cancer Treatment Centers of America combines conventional cancer treatment with non-harmful complimentary approaches, using Naturopathic doctors. In essence, all of the natural supplements discussed in this book are a form of naturopathic medicine.

Like naturopathic medicine, alternative medicine seeks to not harm the patient, and is therefore holistic in nature. Alternative medicine uses non-conventional therapies in treating cancer too, however, they typically fall farther outside of conventional medicine than naturopathic medicine does. An excellent example of a conventional doctor using alternative medicine is Doctor Tullio Simoncini's use of sodium bicarbonate to heal cancer by injecting it into a vein that leads directly to a tumor. Intravenous Vitamin C therapy, Chelation, Hyperthermia and Ozone Therapy are other examples of alternative therapies, and are used by certified doctors, who are operating in an alternative medical context.

Acupuncturists and Eastern medicine also fit under the alternative umbrella. Eastern medicine can be a powerful form of healing and much of it is supported by science. Sadly, the FDA and the cancer industry tend to shrug their shoulders at alternative medicine. Their chief complaint is that alternative therapies are not supported by science. When the Western mindset does not understand something it tends to label it as unscientific and throws the baby out with the bathwater.

Nevertheless, if enough Americans become aware of how Machiavellian chemo and radiation therapy are, then perhaps one day there will be an army of people lobbying Congress, the FDA, and their insurance companies to afford us a safer and more effective option.

Anyhow, most of us are not prepared to face the side effects that come our way in the post treatment period. I felt as though I was always a step or so behind the power curve in understanding exactly what I was supposed to be doing. It was kind of like dancing with a girl the first time and not knowing where to place your hands or feet. However, the naturopathic and alternative doctors that I consulted with showed me where to place my hands and how to get into better step with the music.

Summary

If we decide to do nothing to fight cancer during the post treatment period, we will be at a much higher risk of recurrence. Remember, the worst kinds of recurrence are within the first year after treatment. Even if we do experience a recurrence, it is certain that it will be less severe than if we had done nothing to prevent recurrence in the first place.

To prevent recurrence, it is critical to maintain healthy body ecology. This requires holistic eating and lifestyle habits, including daily exercise and targeted natural supplements, things based on clinical studies that collectively build the body's immune system to resist cancer. All of the holistic antidotes discussed thus far are scientifically based, safe, and invite anyone with cancer to put them into practice.

Notwithstanding the good intentions of doctors and nurses, they typically do not have a treatment plan for most side effects, unless they are extremely serious or life threatening. This means the patient is in the driver's seat as to how well most of their side effects are managed. Some side effects are persistent and difficult to treat because the chemistry of the body has been terribly upset. This means each patient should be aggressive in understanding their side effects and how they can heal from them.

We can talk to ourselves all we want to, and weigh all of the information that we come across, but just thinking about stuff doesn't get the job done. This is where a consult with an expert outside of conventional medicine, might help move the healing ball down the court much farther than it otherwise would. After seeing several naturopathic and alternative doctors, I experienced improvement in most of the areas I sought help in. I am certain they will be able to help you too.

We also have to be prepared to manage complacency. Everyone has to. It goes with the territory. Once we recover and start feeling better, old eating and lifestyle habits come knocking at the door. Do not open that door. If you invite the bad habit back in, then kick it out and start over. Do not stop taking the natural supplements that are clinically proven to resist cancer. It's easy to give up on them when you think you are out of the woods, when you're really not. The point is, once you have cancer you are never out of the woods.

Even if we cannot be perfect in all our habits, any good ones we adapt will place us in the best possible position to live longer with a better quality of life. Finally, stand on the one truth we should all have learned by now, and that is the body is able to heal itself from virtually anything if it is given the right support. So what are you waiting for? Start replacing those bad habits with good ones today!

Notes

1. "Chemotherapy Effects on Organs/Body Systems." Health Encyclopedia University of Rochester Medical Center. http://urmc.rochester.edu/encyclopedia/content.aspx? ContentTypeID=85&ContentID=P07155 (accessed September 23, 2016)

2. Ibid.

3. "Chemo Brain," American Cancer Society, http://www.cancer.org/ treament/treatmentsandsideeffects/physicalsideeffects/chemo-therapyeffects/chemo-brain (accessed September 20, 2016, 1).

4. Cancer Update: Research Update 2002-2003 http://www.eyeson the prize. org /links/researchupdate2002-03.html#feb2002 (accessed September 20, 2016).

5. Mercola, Joseph, MD, "Top 7 Foods To Boost Brain Power," January 15, 2015. http://www.articles.mercola.com/sites/articles/archive/201/ 01/12/top-7- brain- foods.aspx (accessed September 23, 2015.

6. Abdull Ravis AF, Noor NM, "Cruciferous Vegetables: Dietary Phyto chemicals for Cancer Prevention". Asian Pac J Cancer Prev. 2013;1-4(3): 1565-70. http://www.ncbi.nlm.nih.gov/pubmed/23 679237

7. "Cruciferous Vegetables and Cancer Prevention." http://www.cancer.gov/about-cancer/causes-prevention/risk/diet/ cruciferousvegetables-fact-sheet

8. Roxanne Nelson, "Cruciferous Veggies Boost Survival in Breast Cancer Patients," April 2012, http://www.medscape.com/view-article/761792 (accessed August 14, 2016)

9. Feskanich D, Ziegler RG, Michaud DS, et al. Prospective study of fruit and vegetable consumption and risk of lung cancer among men and women. J Natl Cancer Inst. 2000; 92(22):1812-2.

CHAPTER 15

Dealing With Recurrence

For wisdom is better than rubies, and all the things
one may desire cannot be compared with her.
—Proverbs 8:11

Two years had passed while I was under endoscopic and PET scan surveillance, with nothing but negative diagnostics, negative biopsies, and no sign of Barrett's Esophagus. Things were looking pretty encouraging. Every time I saw my Gastroenterologist and Oncologist they would shake their heads in amazement as to the healing I experienced. Other good things occurred as well. The chemo-fog lifted enough for me to reenter the classroom part-time, teaching college math; and I loved it. Unfortunately, life can change as quickly as a thunderstorm rolls in, seemingly out of nowhere. The change I was about to experience would be one of those capricious moments. It caught every one off guard. It seems once you have cancer, life becomes a tricky proposition no matter what.

It was January 19th, 2016, and I had just completed the two-year surveillance endoscopy, when life veered down another rocky road. What sticks in my mind the most that morning is Doctor G. saying, "I've got some bad news for you Joe. A small tumor, 1.5 cm has returned in a location just below the site of the original tumor, and it extends into the cardia, which is the upper part of the stomach. It's time to call Doctor S." Kelly's face was ashen. So was mine. We were both speechless, and other than a few comments, so was the doctor. Getting into a head on collision for a second time is crushing.

Most cancer patients with recurrent disease, be it metastatic or not, do not have the foggiest idea that there exists a large bouquet of alternative therapies available to them. These alternative therapies can be used as complements for any sort of treatment program, thus attacking the cancer from multiple angles. One approach is not exclusive of the other. They can be done in tandem, or in sequence, as the circumstances dictate.

This chapter discusses various options recurrent cancer patients might have in regard to conventional, integrative and alternative medicine, so that they may develop a tangible plan of action should they experience a recurrence.

This chapter also explores a number of other important issues related to recurrence, namely, clinical trials, targeted therapies, cancer stem cells, immunotherapy, early detection cancer blood tests, and alternative cancer centers in the United States that are scarcely known by most people.

Standard Of Care Treatment Options

The Standard Of Care (SOC) for treating cancer is founded primarily on three modes of treatment: chemotherapy, radiation therapy and surgery. The types and amounts of chemo and radiation that may be delivered to a patient have all been extensively tested through clinical trials and approved by the FDA. The doctor has little say in the treatment options. Surgery is considered to be the most important of the three modalities. This is because it can completely remove a tumor, while the other two modes of therapy cannot.

Chemotherapy and radiation therapy are typically used to downgrade the tumor, to help prevent it from spreading, and to make the tumor easier to remove by surgery. Downgrading the tumor also helps reduce the risk of the cancer spreading, as a result of the surgery. So, what does one do if they finish cancer treatment and it comes back? Well, it depends on a lot of factors.

The first key factor is what type of shape the patient is in. If the patient has comorbidities going on, such as severe anemia from chemo, or heart disease, they might not be healthy enough to receive certain additional treatments.

The second key factor is whether the cancer is non-metastatic or metastatic; in other words, how far advanced is the recurrence? There may be treatment options still available in the former case, but not necessarily in the latter one. For instance, as the tumor gets larger it expands into surrounding tissue. It might migrate into areas where radiation or surgery is too dangerous to perform. If the cancer has spread to other areas of the body, creating numerous other tumors, then the level of radiation and chemo required to neutralize these tumors could kill the patient before the therapy does.

What often occurs is that patients are given one modality of treatment in an effort to extend life, not to cure the patient. Although additional chemotherapy might be able to slow a metastatic tumor down, all cancers eventually become resistant to it. In this case, the patient is slowly poisoned to death by the toxic treatment, while the cancer is starving the patient to death. All of these things are why earlier staged cancers are much more treatable.

Third, the treatment for recurrence depends on whether or not the patient has already received the maximum tolerable dose of chemo and radiation, or has had surgery. Since I had already received chemo and radiation, it was not an option for me. Why? It didn't work—that's why the cancer came back. This is why surgery was the only option left.

Fortunately, my cancer was not metastatic. This made me a good candidate for the surgery. Of note, Oncologists cannot offer patients a clinical trial until the patient has failed all components of the SOC established by the FDA for their particular type of cancer.

Aside from the three primary modes of treatment, there are targeted therapies that are available to some patients, particularly Immunotherapy. Immunotherapy is a newer mode of treatment that is still being tested in various trials. Some patients are seeing improved outcomes with Immunotherapy, but it is not yet widely used. Targeted therapies will be discussed in more detail later in this chapter.

If a patient has metastatic cancer, and he or she has failed the three modalities of treatment, and a targeted therapy is not available, their Oncologist might offer them an experimental drug, or a clinical trial. At this point, some might argue that they are grasping at straws, because these later modes are essentially trial and error experiments on humans that have little chance of succeeding.

My Experience

Fortunately, my cancer was not metastatic and the surgery option was still on the cancer treatment roulette table. Regrettably however, if I knew what I know now about alternative therapies and the brutality of the esophagectomy, I might have opted out of the surgery and tried the alternative route first. In the absence of a well thought out back-up plan, I reluctantly went through with the surgery. It was ruthless. Among other things, I suffered a collapsed lobe in both lungs, was on a feeding tube for 11 weeks, and lost 40 pounds. I had other complications that went on for months following treatment, including a serious one that I am still dealing with almost two years post surgery.

I received a dosage of almost 50 Gy—pronounced gray, of absorbed radiation during cancer treatment. The dosage was delivered over the course of five weeks in a very small area of the body. So how much radiation is this? To give you a better idea, let's take a look at Federal mandated safe levels. The International Standard, and Title 10, Part 20 of the Code of Federal Regulations, sets safe exposure limits for those who work with or around radioactive material, including those in nuclear medicine, to be no more than 5,000 mrems over 12 months. Now hold on to your hat. The radiation I received was 1,000 times more radiation exposure than the maximum safe limit. It is astonishing to me that radiation is still being used to treat cancer in the 21st century. Keep in mind that this dosage was delivered in a little over five weeks and in a very narrow area of the body. In comparison, the maximum safe exposure limit is determined by spreading it over the entire area of the body over 12 months. Understanding all of this begs the question: was my recurrence induced by radiation therapy? No one knows for sure, but I have a hunch. I believe it was radiation induced, because the tumor was located just below the site of the original tumor, which had healed—so, that's my take on it, anyway.

Recurrent metastatic esophageal cancer, as is the case with most other metastatic cancers, usually comes with a near term expiration date stamped on the birth certificate. So why is recurrence so dangerous? Tumor cells and stem cells will eventually leak out of the tumor into the lymph nodes and blood. The more advanced the stage the higher the risk of cancer cells getting into the lymph nodes and blood stream. These circulating cells are very difficult to treat. They can spread to other areas of the body without being detected by current diagnostic tests. Cancer cells learn how to resist all types of chemo drugs if given enough time. The cells that survive treatment are typically ones that developed a resistance to the treatment. If they come back they usually do so with a vengeance. This is why chemotherapeutic drugs have such a dreadful track record of curing people of cancer. Yet, most cancer patients, like myself, falsely believe the chemo can cure us.

Anyhow, I had something else that worked against me. Something I didn't realize until later. It had to do with not fully understanding the Ketogenic Diet, and because of this, my effort backfired. I tried to follow a semi-Ketogenic Diet. I cut out all sugar but did not cut the carbohydrates down enough. I also ate too much protein, including cheese. Doing a half-baked Ketogenic Diet ranks at the top of the list of bad ideas. Much to my chagrin, this ill-conceived idea turned into a disaster. By the time the tumor was removed, four weeks later, it had grown from 1.5 to 4.3 cm, making it a Stage 3, and I also had a metastatic lymph node in the local region. So what happened? I didn't know enough about the Ketogenic Diet to understand that it was imperative to monitor blood sugar and ketone levels to determine if the diet was working, and that the protein casein found in dairy products promotes cancer growth, nor did I know about methionine. I would have been much better off if I had simply gone back to the original cancer diet that I put myself on prior to chemo-radiation, because it was strikingly similar to the Hybrid Cancer Diet discussed in Chapter 7. The original tumor shrank form 4 cm to 1.5 cm, allowing treatment to be more effective. The exact reverse happened the second time around, even down to the numbers being the same but reversed. If there is anything to learn from this, it is that the patient has a lot of power to affect the growth of the tumor prior to entering treatment. When cancer patients do not know this truth they miss a tremendous opportunity to impact their outcome. Please do not do what I did, but learn from it. Although I butchered the Ketogenic Diet, I am convinced that the other holistic things I did during the post treatment period prevented recurrence for two years, and helped contain the recurrence to the local area.

Clinical Trials

If a patient fails the SOC their oncologist can refer them to a clinical trial for their type of cancer. Clinical Trials are helpful for establishing new treatment approaches, but very few of them ever make it to market. Some patients can benefit from a clinical trial, but most do not. To be clear, very few metastatic patients survive a clinical trial. I was offered a clinical trial following the surgery because I was in a high-risk category for recurrence.

I found an esophageal cancer clinical trial that momentarily caught my attention, except that it included a double-blind placebo group. In this type of clinical trial, one group of patients receive a fake drug, a placebo, and another group receive the test drug, and neither the patients nor the researchers know who receives what. Suffice to say, I wasn't ready to submit my body to a trial and error experiment for the advancement of pharmacological science—someone else is welcome to my admission ticket.

Targeted Therapies

Targeted therapies use drugs or other substances that specifically target cancer in ways that attempt to minimize harm to healthy cells. For instance, exploiting the metabolic characteristics of cancer using nutritional therapy is a targeted natural therapy. Using drugs that exploit certain genetic processes within a cancer cell is another from of targeted therapy. Scientists are also working on gene-editing techniques that can reverse inherited genes that are flawed or ones that have mutated into a cancer causing form. One of the most promising targeted therapies is called Immunotherapy. It is science that has been around since the 1970's that trumpeted a new era of effective cancer therapy to be just around the corner—but it never materialized.

Immunotherapy uses various drugs that can promote cancer cell death, block a cancer cell's ability to divide, inhibit a tumor from forming new blood vessels, and even activate the body's immune system to attack the cancer. The later one—I believe, holds the greatest promise of finding a substantial cure for cancer, and it will be discussed in more detail later in this section.

According to the National Cancer Institute, Immunotherapy exploits a number of biological mechanisms in the body using monoclonal antibodies, cytokines, therapeutic vaccines [such as Dendritic Cell Therapy], the bacterium Bacillus Calmet-Guérin, cancer-killing viruses, gene therapy, and adoptive T-cell transfer[1] [CAR-T-cell Therapy].

The cancer industry and the government have been over promising major breakthroughs in cancer for decades, however in the area of immunotherapy they have accomplished some improved outcomes. The most recent generation of immunotherapy drugs are extending life in certain types of cancers, namely non-Hodgkin's Lymphoma and Leukemia.

An example of a successful outcome using Immunotherapy is with former President Jimmy Carter. In 2015, President Carter announced that he was fighting metastatic melanoma that had spread to his liver and brain. Doctors first treated him surgically by removing a tumor from the liver. Then he received four rounds of chemo and radiation therapy directed at spots on his brain. Subsequently, he entered into a clinical trial and received an investigational drug called Pembrolizumab, also known as Keytrudra. This drug has since been approved by the FDA and is in wide usage. Pembrolizumab is a monoclonal antibody that binds to a receptor on cancer cells allowing the body's immune system to destroy the cancer. This drug is also being used on advanced non-small cell lung cancer (NSCLC) patients.

President Carter responded to the treatment and his cancer went into remission. Other than President Carter, only a small group of people in the trial responded to the drug[2]—the rest of them died.

Immunotherapy drugs are not unlike other chemo drugs and come with serious side effects. Cancer can adapt to Immunotherapy drugs just like they can with off the shelf chemo agents. There is also a serious risk that these drugs may trigger an autoimmune response, resulting in the immune system attacking normal cells and organs and causing potentially debilitating side effects and even death. According to the American Academy of Dermatology,

> Targeted therapy has been shown to extend life in many patients with advanced melanoma, but the effect is short-lived, as patients typically experience a recurrence of the disease. Although immunotherapy works for fewer individuals, it provides a more long-term response when it does work.[3]

There you have it. The latest generation of Immunotherapy drugs might work in a limited fashion for some, but not for most others.

Another targeted therapy that is gaining wider use is preventive vaccines that attack virus related cancers. For example, the human papillomavirus (HPV) is the most common sexually transmitted virus in

Western countries and can cause cervical, genital, anal, and oropharyngeal cancers. The vaccines developed for HPV have proven to be very effective in preventing cancer.

There is also a vaccine to prevent Hepatitis B, which causes liver cancer. Although this vaccine can help prevent cancer, it was not very effective when used with a group of cancer patients in a Phase III clinical trial. It only prolonged life by an average of four-months.[4]

In comparison to pharmacological Immunotherapy, less harmful alternative medicine Immunotherapy has been studied and successfully used in clinical settings in Europe for a number of years. One of these therapies is called Dendritic Cell Therapy (DCT), which is an Immunotherapy that is similar to a vaccine. DCT will be discussed in detail shortly.

Stem Cells

Cancer stem cells are a special type of cell that every tumor produces. At some point after a tumor forms cancer stem cells and tumor cells their way into the lymph nodes and blood. Cancer stem cells can disguise themselves as normal cells, just like tumor cells can, allowing them to evade the body's immune system. During chemo and radiation both cancer tumor and stem cells mutate into more drug and radiation resistant strains. Both types of cancer cells can become dormant and circulate throughout the body indefinitely, unless something triggers the immune system to target them as pathogens. The stem cells are more dangerous than the tumor cells because they possess the DNA imprint to regenerate a new tumor anywhere in the body. This section will therefore speak directly to the circulating cancer stem cells.

Most patients in remission do not have an inkling of how dangerous cancer stem cells are to their long-term survival. This is because doctors don't know how to effectively kill them, other than to throw more chemo at the patient. Current treatment protocols typically require the patient to receive additional chemo, usually a different type than they first received, knowing that their remaining cancer cells have developed some level of resistance to the drugs that were used. This of course is one of the reasons why some of the cancer cells survived the chemo or radiation in the first place. A lack of understanding in how to expel circulating cancer stem cells explains why there is such a high rate of death among recurrent cancer patients.

The process on how a stem cell reactivates a new tumor, and why it picks one place in the body to regenerate versus another place, is not well understood. Aside from this, circulating cancer stem cells are extremely difficult for the body's immune system to identify, let alone destroy. They disguise themselves as normal cells. Even more alarming, some tumors are able to disable the kill switches on pathogen killing white blood cells. The combination of all of these factors, as well as others, explains why most people who get recurrent cancer will die.

A person in remission needs to have some sense of what they need to do to keep their cancer in remission. Understanding cancer stem cells and options on how to treat them is important, but equally important is getting a grasp on what caused the cancer in the first place. To complicate matters, the patient in remission most likely received the standard of care maximum dose treatment protocol, and now has a body ecology that is in worse shape than it was before the tumor presented. The answer, according to many in alternative medicine, is the whole body needs to be treated and repaired before it will be able to defend itself from a recurrence. They type of treatment they recommend involves detoxification, nutritional therapy, exercise, low stress environment, good sleep, targeted natural substances and therapies—and least not, a therapeutic approach to target circulating cancer stem cells.

In sum, two of the biggest roadblocks to preventing recurrence are how to deal with the elusive drug resistant cancer stems cells and how to rebuild a severely damaged immune system.

It's now time to take a look at several novel alternative Immunotherapies that can target and kill circulating stems cells. These therapies are only available at a few medical centers in the Untied States and they are not widely known or understood. So are you ready? Let's roll up our sleeves and press into some exciting new information.

Several Novel Immunotherapies

Dendritic Cell Therapy

One of the most promising immunotherapies is Dendritic Cell Therapy (DCT), which found its way to the United States from Germany over two decades ago. DCT has proven to be very safe and effective in many contexts, but unfortunately the United States has been very slow in fully adapting it. One might ask, why? I am not entirely sure why, but suspect that part of the reason is that DCT is not a copyrightable pharmacological solution.

Dendritic cells are specialized white blood cells that are produced in the bone marrow. Their primary function is to identify and capture pathogens and then present them to killer T-cells in the lymph nodes. The T-cells then go on a search and destroy mission for the newly identified pathogen. DCT uses the body's white blood cells to create a vaccine that will trigger an immune response that can accurately identify and kill cancer cells. Remember, cancer cells disguise themselves as normal cells, and they can also emit proteins that can disable certain elements of the immune system. DCT allows our immune cells to accurately identify cancer cells as pathogens.

A number of different types of DC therapy are being studied and used in clinical settings. In this section, we will examine two types of DCT therapy, one that uses a virus to help stimulate an immune response and one that does not. Both approaches come with relatively few side effects, especially the one that does not use a virus.

DCT has been used to treat cancer in Europe, particularly in Germany, for decades. Although it has been studied in the United States for several decades, it has not gained wide acceptance. One form of DCT that was popularized in Germany is now being used on a limited basis in the United States. It uses a poultry virus called the Newcastle Disease Virus (NDV). NDV is not harmful to humans but can infect cancer cells, which will then stimulate an immune response through the dendritic cells. To create the vaccine, blood is drawn from the patient and a sophisticated process is used to harvest cancer cells and a special type of white blood cell, called a dendritic cell. They culture the NDV with the patient's dendritic cells to create something similar to a vaccine. The vaccine is injected into the patient to stimulate an immune response. The FDA approved the first NDV vaccine in 2010, called Dendreon's Provenge, which is used against prostate cancer. Several improved DC vaccines are currently in clinical trials with the expectation they will produce improved outcomes and ultimately be approved by the FDA. In certain cases patients with a cancer other than prostate cancer can apply for a compassionate use waiver by the FDA, which permits someone's blood to be sent to a lab in Germany to produce the NDV-DC vaccine, and then shipped back to the United States.

Another type of DC therapy called Immune Support Therapy (IST), doesn't use a virus to infect the cancer cell but relies entirely on the patient's own immune cells. Clinical success rates are being reported as high as 80 percent for IST. This type of approach is called Adaptive Cell Transfer because it collects the patient's own immune cells to create a vaccine. The dendritic cells are loaded up with antigens that have been exposed to the peptides that are specific to their cancer and are then able to present these identifiers to the body's T cells. Once the T cells get the new information an immune response is initiated. IST does have some mild side effects that come as a result of stimulating an immune response, which include a low-grade fever, headache, fatigue, chills, or a mild skin rash at the sight of the tumor that may last from three to 14 days. These side effects are minor compared to current Immunotherapy drugs, including NDV-DC therapy. Although alternative IST has found its way to the United States, it is only offered by a very limited number of doctors in states that have patient friendly experimental cancer treatment laws.

IST and other safer immunotherapies are offered by Issels Immuno-Oncology and the Cancer Center for Healing. Both are located in California and are discussed in an upcoming section on alternative cancer centers.

CAR-T-Cell Therapy

Instead of using dendritic cells, CAR-T-cell therapy is an immunotherapy that creates a vaccine out of a patient's T cells. T cells are a special type of pathogen killing white blood cell. The FDA approved CAR-T-cell therapy in October 2017 for use with various blood related cancers. Many hope this therapy will be effective in treating blood related cancers in children.

CAR-T-cell therapy genetically modifies a receptor on a T-cell that will allow it to recognize and attach to a specific antigen or protein on the surface of a cancer cell. An unfortunate aspect of this approach is that they have to destroy much of the patient's normal T-cells before they administer the vaccine. The injection is preceded by a lymopho-depleting chemo regimen. The side effects can be serious. According to the American Cancer Society's web page on "CAR T-cell Side Effects,"

Serious side effects can include very high fevers and dangerously low blood pressure in the days after it's given. Other serious side effects include neurotoxicity or changes in the brain that cause confusion, seizures, or severe headaches. Some patients have also developed serious infections, low blood cell counts and a weakened immune system. These side effects can be life threatening . . . ."

So this is where the hundreds of billions of dollars spent on cancer research over the last fifty years have gotten us. Let's now take a look at a novel alternative approach that uses DNA testing and epigenetics in a way that helps the body restore damaged immune functions.

Epigenetic Therapy

Epigenetics is the science of how differences or aberrations in cells can turn genes on or off. For example, if inherited genes, viruses, toxins or chemo and radiation disrupt normal gene processes, genes can malfunction and promote cancer, heart conditions, mental illness, diabetes and other degenerative diseases. The premise of the healing approach in epigenetics is to discover what conditions caused the cancer in the first place, and then to reverse or restore these conditions to a healthy state.

Epigenetics requires extensive testing of a patient's DNA and body ecology. Once a detailed biochemical analysis is performed, the doctor develops a unique treatment plan that uses predominantly alternative and holistic techniques, and is tailored to each patient's biological profile. This approach can also employ herbal detoxification and nutritional therapy to restore the cellular biology to a healthier condition. Included with the DNA testing are other tests that evaluate types and levels of chemical toxicity, including cell radiation load. Doctors who practice this niche area of alternative medicine are experts in nutrition, biochemistry and epigenetics and can unlock the mechanisms of all sorts of degenerative conditions and diseases.

Epigenetic Therapy is potentially an excellent adjunct to another therapy such as IST, or any other kind of conventional or alternative treatment plan. In fact, this is exactly the treatment protocol I started as I finished the second edition of this book. Epigenetics is a very complicated science, and to my knowledge, there are not a lot of doctors providing this service to cancer patients in the United States.

Alternative cancer medicine contends that cancer stem cells remain in the body for years after a patient enters remission, especially for those with late stage cancers. The higher the stage the more likely it is that the tumor has released radiation and chemo resistant stem cells into the blood. A cancer in remission is certainly something to rejoice in, but doing so should be tempered with a sober awareness that a serious risk of recurrence remains, unless a post treatment plan is developed that intentionally restores the immune system and targets the cancer stem cells.

Let's next look at some important early detection cancer tests, and understand their actual levels of sensitivity. Some of these tests may very well help save your life, if implemented aggressively as part of a post remission treatment plan. Remember, the earlier the detection, the easier it is to treat, and the higher the survival.

Early Detection Cancer Tests

Other than not going on a vegan centric cancer diet, or having an alternative cancer treatment option in place, I also wish I had not relied so heavily on the PET scan and endoscopic surveillance alone, to detect recurrence. Little did I know that there are extremely sensitive early detection cancer blood tests that are available in the United States and Europe.

ONCOblot Test: The ONCOblot test is an extremely sensitive ultra-early cancer detection test. It is classified as a secondary prevention test because it detects cancer very early when it is not as dangerous and is easier to treat. When cancer cells divide they release a unique protein into the blood, the ENOX2 marker, but normal cells do not. This test measures the microscopic load of ENOX2 in the blood. This test exhibits an unparalleled sensitivity of 97.3 percent.[6] It can measure a tumor down to about 1 to 2 mm, which is about 4/100 of an inch, roughly the size of a pin head. In comparison, a mammogram detects a tumor at about 7.5 mm, or roughly 30/100 of an inch, and a PET scan to about 5 mm, which is 20/100 of an inch, but only with very aggressive cancers.[7] If it is not a very aggressive form of cancer, the PET scan has difficulty detecting tumors that are smaller that 10 mm, 40/100 of an inch.[8]

The ONCOblot test can pick up as few as 2 million cancer cells in the blood or lymphatic system before a tumor has formed.[9] It can detect more than one cancer and identify their tissues of origin, and cancers of unknown primary (CUP), also known as occult primary tumor. CUP cancers are typically metastatic cancers that are active in some area of the body other than from where they originated. For instance, breast cancer cells can spread to the lungs and form a tumor there, but cancer markers identify them as breast cancer cells with an unknown location.

Even more impressive, this test has a false positive rate of less than 1 percent, and can detect Stage 0 cancer, such as DCIS, which is a localized breast cancer.[10] Moreover, the ONCOblot provides an excellent second step test in validating the presence of active cancer cells when other tests such as High PSA, PET scans, biopsies, and mammograms are suspicious or inconclusive.[11] The ONCOblot test provides excellent diagnostic support in post surgery or other post cancer treatment scenarios to validate the presence or absence of active cancer cells. This latter case is of tremendous value to patients like myself who completed the standard of care treatment for esophageal cancer and were offered additional chemotherapy prophylactically, without even knowing whether any cancer is still present. Patients who complete radiation, chemo and surgery are terribly compromised. The last thing the patient wants to do is receive an unnecessary round of chemo, since it can create an environment that promotes recurrence.

The ENOX 2 protein has the ability to pass through the blood-brain barrier. This provides an additional diagnostic indicator for those with active brain cancer, as well as an early detection test for those under surveillance. Sadly, insurance companies do not currently pay for this groundbreaking diagnostic test. This test costs around 1,000 dollars, depending on the cancer center that orders it.

The ENOX2 protein is detected in the following cancers:

Bladder	Non-Small cell	Squamous Cell
Breast	Lung Small cell	Follicular Thyroid
Cervical	Lymphoma	Papillary Thyroid
Colorectal	Melanoma	Testicular (Germ
Endometrial	Mesothelioma	Cell)
Esophageal	Myeloma	Uterine
Gastric	Ovarian	
Hepatocellular	Pancreatic	
Kidney	Prostate	
Leukemia	Sarcoma	

I was offered a six-month course of Herceptin following surgery because of the high risk of recurrence associated with the presence of a metastatic lymph node. Herceptin is a newer targeted cancer therapy, initially approved exclusively for breast cancer. In 2011, the FDA approved its use for metastatic esophageal adenocarcinoma and gastric cancer. It is a monoclonal antibody that interferes with the receptor on cancer cells and inhibits their ability to divide into new cells. Herceptin is used as an option in early stage breast cancer, and also for late stage recurrence where it might prolong life by a few months or even longer. For esophageal and gastric cancer it can be used in the same context as breast cancer. According to Memorial Sloan Kettering Cancer Center, however, it might be effective initially in some esophageal cancer patients but most develop resistance to it and the cancer progresses.[12] In short, it has a poor track record with esophageal cancer, so I was not excited about taking it. I asked Doctor O. if he had a blood test to detect cancer markers for my tumor. He said, "No, there are no such markers for esophageal cancer." I asked, "Do you mean to say that I would be taking this chemo drug prophylactically, even though I may not have any active cancer cells in my blood?" He replied, "Yes, you have a very dangerous cancer. It might be better to treat you with something rather than doing nothing. In your situation Herceptin would be more experimental. I am sorry, but I do not have anything else to offer you."

I understood his point entirely. I then asked, "Please tell me if there is a tumor sensitivity test available for Herceptin and esophageal cancer?" He replied, "No, I am sorry, but there isn't." I sensed his frustration for me, that there was nothing else he could offer other than a clinical trial, which I later turned down too. I thought to myself, "Throwing wet spaghetti noodles on the wall to see if they stick is not for me." It also entreats the question, "What incentive is there in taking a drug that chemically damages the body with little certainty it will work?" The risk to reward profile for Herceptin was not inspiring.

At this point, I decided it would be better to pay out of pocket for an alternative/integrative cancer treatment program. Shortly after seeing Doctor O., I scheduled a four-week program with EuroMed Foundation in Phoenix, Arizona and purchased my round trip airfare. I had several extensive phone consults with their chief Administrator, Doctor D. He was detailed and thorough, and carefully answered all of my questions. He also explained,

> We have treated a number of late stage esophageal cancer patients in past years with limited success, but have recently developed a protocol that is proving to be very promising. Unfortunately, most of our cancer patients are later stage cancers that have failed traditional treatment, and they are in really bad condition. Even under those circumstances, we are extending life in many of our patients for years not months.

EuroMed offers a comprehensive treatment program. It is tailored to the needs of each patient. At the minimum, it typically includes detoxification, holistic nutrition, intravenous immune therapy, and Insulin Potentiated Therapy (IPT), also known as fractionalized chemo. IPT is held by many in alternative therapy to be a much safer and more effective than low dose chemotherapy. It employs a basket of two or more chemo drugs that work synergistically against the cancer. Patients are required to fast for at least 12 hours before the therapy to lower their blood sugar, which is intended to make the insulin portion of the therapy more effective. Patients receive an injection of insulin right before the low dose chemo is given to "potentiate" the cancer cells to take in more chemo. Patients experience few side effects because the drugs are administered in a very low dose. I encountered a number of arguments by conventional cancer researchers and doctors that refute IPT as an effective therapy, but substantial clinical evidence suggests otherwise.

EuroMed's program is outpatient, Monday through Friday, and costs roughly 5,000 or more dollars per week depending on how much of the program the patient participates in. This cost seems reasonable for what they provide, particularly after I discovered that similar centers were more on the order of 6,000 to 7,000 dollars per week. As a side note, most centers require patients to sign up for their entire treatment protocol. In some cases, centers are willing to work with patients and get costs down to the 3,000 to 5,000 dollar range by dropping some of the complementary treatments. Even though the chemo agents that are used in IPT are all off the shelf and FDA approved, insurance companies refuse to pay for it. So I asked, "Why?" My insurance company told me that IPT is considered an experimental treatment. Sadly, IPT and many other effective or helpful alternative/integrative treatments have been consigned to the cancer therapy leper colony.

As it is with most other alternative/integrative treatment centers, EuroMed provides a list of hotels in the local area that offer discounts to their patients. EuroMed is staffed by state certified doctors, nurses and other practitioners. The program can last four or more weeks depending on the severity of the disease and the condition of the patient. Numerous people share their testimonies of amazing outcomes on the EuroMed website. Credible patient testimonies and reviews are an extremely important part of the decision process.

EuroMed's treatment would be prophylactic, just as Doctor O. recommended. It would start May 1, only two and a half months following the surgery. By the way, everything I was doing in the alternative arena was being bounced off my primary care doctor. Be careful not to cut your primary doctors out of the equation because they provide a very important element in your overall healing and welfare.

EuroMed was terribly concerned about my high-grade tumor with lymph node involvement and did not want to wait for a chemo sensitivity test that needed to be sent overseas. They claimed that they had developed a very effective basket of chemo agents that were working well on their esophageal cancer patients, so it wasn't worth the risk of waiting for an overseas test to come back.

Instead, I had the ONCOblot test and the results were negative. However, my Oncologist and EuroMed advised that I treat this type of cancer prophylactically. As it happens, I was in such bad shape from the surgery that I was not able to travel anywhere. I had lost 40 pounds and I was still on a feeding tube, having to feed myself multiple times a day with liquids from a large syringe like device. I could only take sips of water, no more than one ounce per hour. I was on the feeding tube for 11 weeks. When I was able to eat again it was mostly liquid or soft food for almost two years because of complications from the surgery. Since I was in no shape for a treatment center, I received additional nutritional counseling and explored some safe natural supplement therapies available locally, such as high dose intravenous Vitamin C, Artesunate and oxygen therapy.

Many believe high dose Vitamin C bolsters the immune system and relieves oxidative stress, potentially killing cancer cells.[13] It would be almost 15 months following the surgery that I was strong enough to enter into a month long alternative therapy program.

<u>The Greece Tests:</u> The Greece Tests are a series of cancer blood tests offered by the Research Genetic Cancer Centre (R.G.C.C.) at overseas labs. Any doctor in the United States can draw your blood and ship it overseas via an R.G.C.C. representative organization in Texas.

The Greece Tests offer excellent diagnostic specificity for early detection, characterizing cancer, and developing more effective targeted therapies. These tests are best used in an integrative treatment scenario where other diagnostics such as PET scans and cancer markers play an important role.

The out of pocket cost of these exams is between 500 to 3,000 dollars, depending on the test. The URL is: gcc-group.com.

> <u>The Greece Tests can do the following:</u>
> 1) Identify cancer cell markers relative to a specific type of malignancy, and the immunophenotype of leukemias and lymphomas.
> 2) Assess the presence of circulating tumor cells and any positive circulating stem cells, including their concentration.
> 3) Measure the sensitivity/resistance of your cancer cells to 53 cytotoxic drugs, 48 monoclonal antibodies, and 46 natural substances and plant extracts, which can be used as a targeted therapy by a Naturopathic or Alternative doctor. Some of these biologic substances include Intenzyme Forte, Poly-MVA, Laetrile, Melatonin, Vitamin D3 and Quecertin.
> 4) Identify genes that can be potentially used in targeted therapy.[14]

<u>Cancer Markers:</u> Cancer Markers are blood tests that measure the level of specific proteins or genes in tissue, blood, or other bodily fluids that may indicate precancer or cancer activity. They do not detect stem cells. Many, but not all cancers have markers, some of which can be targeted with drugs. An elevated tumor marker level is not enough information to diagnose cancer. It only suggests the presence of cancer. If cancer is confirmed through other diagnostic methods, then tumor markers may help determine if the cancer is growing or regressing. In some cancers, markers can be used to evaluate the tumor's stage, assess the effectiveness of treatment and assist with prognosis. Cancer markers are also effectively used in post treatment surveillance. Although cancer markers are helpful diagnostic tools they are best used with other diagnostic tests. Some cancers, like esophageal and stomach cancer do not have specific tumor markers.

Cologuard: The Cologuard is an early detection colorectal cancer test and works by detecting precancerous or cancerous cells as they pass through the stool. Test kits are ordered directly from the factory and shipped UPS to the patient. The test includes instructions on how to use the kit and ship it back. The results of the test are sent directly to the patient's doctor. Cologuard does not replace surveillance or diagnostic colonoscopies. It provides another means of detecting cancer early. It is proven to be 92 percent accurate in detecting colon cancer cells and 69 percent in precancerous cells.[15] This test is expensive compared to traditional colorectal tests. Yet, the FDA reported Cologuard to be more accurate than the fecal immunochemical test (FIT), with an accuracy of 72 percent.[16] Other tests used to detect colorectal cancer are the guaiac-based fecal occult blood test (gFOBT) test, and Stool DNA test (sDNA).[17]

Prostate-specific Antigen (PSA) Blood Test: The PSA test is one of the most widely used early detection tests for prostate cancer. It is not a definitive test and requires other diagnostics to prove the existence of cancer. Most men do not realize how inaccurate it can be and are at risk of gaining a false sense of security because their number looks good. Most men who have a PSA below 4 do not have cancer, yet it is only 85 percent accurate. Men with a PSA between 4 to 10 have a 25 percent chance of having cancer; and if the PSA is over 10 the risk of cancer is about 50 percent.[18]

PAP Test: The PAP test, also called a PAP smear, is an early detection test for cervical cancer that has been widely used for many years. A PAP smear is routinely taken of the cervical area during an annual physical exam and sent to the lab for analysis. There is a paucity of clear information as to its accuracy. Some opinions on health websites report accuracy ranging between 70 to 80 percent and so do many doctors' offices.

Nevertheless, a group of eight doctors published a report that examined sensitivity (the true positive rate), and specificity (the true negative rate) of the PAP test. By the way, the true negative rate is used to determine false positives. For example, a true negative rate of 86 to 100 percent means the false positive rate is between 0 to 14 percent. These doctors performed a systematic review of 97 different studies on the accuracy of PAP tests and concluded that sensitivity and specificity varied widely between studies. In other words, these tests are prone to error. They also reported that 85 of the 97 studies were biased and therefore inconclusive. The 12 remaining studies were deemed unbiased and were evaluated separately. Their findings were astounding in that the sensitivity of PAP smears ranged a whopping 30 to 87 percent. False positives ranged from 0 to 14 percent. They concluded, "Most studies of the conventional PAP test are severely biased: The best estimates suggest that it is only moderately accurate and does not achieve concurrently high sensitivity and specificity."[19]

Alternative Cancer Treatment as an Option

Although a comprehensive review of alternative cancer treatment centers is outside the scope of this chapter, let's take a look at a number of alternative centers that are producing improved outcomes, particularly in cases where patients failed conventional treatment. These centers have all gained a good reputation and are staffed with certified doctors and nurses, with therapies that are research based, and they have a proven track record of success. In fact, what I discovered surprised me. My predisposition was that such centers only existed in other countries with more flexible alternative treatment laws, such as Mexico, Spain, or Germany. This is not the case. There are a number of excellent alternative cancer centers within the United States, but they are not well advertised. Many of these centers are also integrative, meaning they offer a safer conventional approach to treating cancer, such as IPT, which is a high frequency, low dose chemo approach, also referred to as fractionalized chemo.

Alternative cancer centers get a hard knock by many accusing them of selling snake oil to unwitting victims. Certainly scams exist. However, victimhood lurks in the shadows of those who tend to buy used cars without first looking under the hood. Reputable alternative cancer centers prove easy to identify with a diligent screening process. Before we look at a screening process, let's discuss alternative cancer centers in general.

The best centers produce a lot of satisfied cash-paying customers who are happy to refer others to the same center, and who are also happy to provide written or video testimonies of their experience. Few people will take the time to provide a personal testimony unless they are convinced their testimony may help others. This means the person providing the testimony perceives they experienced a more successful outcome than conventional treatment could offer. To that point, defective products and services do not survive long in the cash paying alternative-cancer therapy market. It is a difficult industry to break into without the support of the insurance companies. However, many insurance companies pay for much of the blood work, as long as the patient files a claim for reimbursement.

Almost every center I spoke to required cash up front on a week-to week basis. The good thing about this is that the patient has an opportunity to withdraw from the program anytime they are not happy with it. Some centers are also integrative and combine alternative therapies like hyperthermia, with low dose radiation therapy, or low dose chemotherapy using insulin-potentiated therapy (IPT). It also appears that most people who enter into an alternative treatment facility are first and foremost, desperate. They are at the end of their rope.

Needless to say, most people remain hesitant to undertake an alternative center, particularly if their insurance does not cover it. Paying out of pocket is a significant roadblock for many, who either lack the funds to do so, or have the funds but lack the confidence to stray outside of conventional treatment.

Another roadblock is that alternative cancer therapies are not part of the public discussion. The alternative cancer therapy approach exists in its own subculture, isolated from the mainstream media, and scorned by the conventional cancer industry—sort of like a harshly treated weakling in a large litter of puppies. They don't measure up to the societal norm. The average patient does not mingle in holistic healing circles and is therefore uninformed. Medical science is complicated to begin with let alone understanding something beyond the pale of medical orthodoxy. This is why few people are interested in an alternative cancer therapy if you mention it to them. I know this first hand. They are afraid of something they know little about, so they ask for the opinion of trusted family members or friends, who work in traditional medicine, or they ask their doctor, all of whom may possess incomplete knowledge in regard to the safe therapies that are available today. Most do not even understand that these alternative therapies can be easily integrated as an adjunct to a conventional treatment program. Consequently, the uninformed patient becomes fearful and exorcizes the whole idea. No one is to blame for this. It is simply a reality of the culture's psyche. Alternative cancer treatment exists in a parallel universe that requires an open mind to learn about what it might offer. Therefore, it seems appropriate to point out that there are prerequisite conditions that enable a person to leap across the chasm of indecision into the dimension of alternative or integrative cancer therapy. One is desperation. The second is sufficient funds. And the third is knowledge.

For alternative and or integrative therapies to be an adjunct to a conventional treatment program, there needs to be buy in from all of the doctors involved. This might be problematic for some conventional doctors, due to their mistrust of alternative medicine. An excellent compromise might be to find an Integrative doctor, who combines alternative therapies with conventional ones. In some cases, an Integrative doctor may not offer radiation or surgery, but instead offer low dose chemotherapy, along with various alternative therapies. To be honest, if I had a chance to do treatment over again, I believe I would go with this approach. All of the alternative treatment centers I interviewed were treating patients who had predominantly failed conventional treatment. It seems very few cancer patients go the alternative route first. Still, there is nothing to preclude a patient from working with an alternative or naturopathic doctor while going through conventional therapy. In most cases, the patient will not be able to overlap both conventional and alternative therapies at the same time. While going through conventional treatment, I used naturopathic doctors to assist in fortifying my immune system, and in identifying natural substances that resist cancer and reduce the side effects of chemo and radiation.

I kept my Oncologist informed of the natural substances I was taking and he had no problem with it. As a side note, alternative and integrative therapies are purposed to kill the cancer while causing the least possible harm to the patient.

So what rubric does one use to find an alternative cancer center? It is paramount to read and understand what the center reveals on their website in regard to their therapies, the science behind their therapies, and any patient reviews and testimonies that back up their claims. Second, it is vital to speak to one of their doctors, nurses or administrators and ask them a number of pointed questions and allow them to explain why their therapies might give you a better chance of surviving compared to your present course of treatment. If possible, these consults should be done in person so that you may also tour their facility. A Skype session can fill the gap too, if travel is too expensive. Third, understand the costs and how you intend to pay for them. Fourth, prepare a number of questions that need to be answered to your satisfaction, to give you enough confidence to make an informed decision, one way or the other. Remember, knowledge is power and due diligence begets confidence in making the right decision. We better get it right the first time, since most of us do not have a lot of time, money or immune system capacity to tinker around with an ineffective treatment pathway.

It's time to explore a number of good questions to ask when researching an alternative cancer center.

1. Is the center certified by the state, do they hire only licensed medical staff, and do they display their state license in their office?

2. Is the facility clean?

3. Are they following careful hygiene practices, such as wearing gloves and not reusing instruments?

4. Is the staff professionally dressed, courteous, and competent?

5. Have any of the doctors been sued for malpractice and why? Don't rush to judgment but understand why. Doctors are sometimes unfairly charged with circumstances outside their control. They might also get caught in the emotional crosshairs of a grieving family.

6. What therapies do they offer for your type of cancer and are they scientifically based approaches supported by published studies in medical journals? Peer reviewed material is desirable. FDA approved procedures are a plus. Do they integrate any conventional treatments with alternative ones? An integrative approach to treating cancer is an excellent way to go for someone not completely sold on alternative therapy.

There is no silver bullet to killing cancer. However, a comprehensive approach from different angles provides the best opportunity to substantially extend life.

7. Are there credible patient testimonies of successful outcomes available on their website or YouTube, especially for your type of cancer? Patients with less common cancers like ovarian, esophageal, laryngeal, brain and stomach, are less attended at these centers. Cancers with higher rates of incidence, such as breast, lung, and prostate are more likely to be represented in the patient testimony section of their website.

8. Do they have statistics on treatment outcomes for your particular

cancer? In many cases they do not have extensive records because many people fly in from another area to get treated, then leave, and never follow up. Are you ready to look at a number of centers?

Alternative Cancer Treatment Centers

All of the treatment centers I listed are cash only and can cost as much as 4,000 to 8,000 dollars per week, depending on the type of treatment offered. I studied their websites and interviewed each center as part of the screening process. A number of centers did not make my final list, even though I researched over 30 facilities offering some form of alternative or integrative cancer therapy. That is not to say that other credible alternative treatment centers in the United State do not exist. Please do your own research and compare what you find to my list, before making a decision. The centers on my list all offer viable options to potentially extend life even after failing conventional treatment. They are not listed in any special order other than to say they are credible, professional, and have excellent patient testimonies to back them up. EuroMed is one of the first ones I was impressed with, so I listed them first.

1. **EuroMed Foundation**: Located in Phoenix, Arizona. EuroMed offers a holistic and integrative approach to cancer treatment. They offer IPT (low dose chemotherapy), along with various natural approaches to healing, such as detoxification, nutritional therapy, natural substance intravenous therapy, such as high dose Vitamin C, Hyperthermia, Ozone Therapy, PEMF (pulsed electro-magnetic therapy), and a homeopathic immune modulator called the George Protocol. They have been successfully treating patients well over a decade. Their website hosts numerous positive testimonies from patients. The URL is: www.euro-med.us

2. **An Oasis of Healing Alternative Cancer Center**: Located in Mesa, Arizona. It offers a whole range of holistic and alternative treatment protocols, which are very similar to EuroMed. They specialize in treating cancer with detoxification, nutrition and fasting, IPT, intravenous Vitamin C and oxidative therapies, such as Ozone Therapy, and Infrared Heat Therapy. This is a smaller cancer center with a very low patient to nurse ratio, allowing more individualized

220

care. With over 12 years of cancer treatment experience, they have accumulated extensive credibility in treating cancer. Their website has a number of patient testimonies who experienced excellent outcomes. URL is: www.anoasisofhealing.com

3. **Cancer Center For Healing:** Located in Irvine, California. This center offers a wide array of holistic and alternative therapies, much like the previous two centers mentioned, including nutrition and exercise. This center also specializes in the R.G.C.C. (Research Genetic Cancer Centre) Greece tests and targeted natural substance therapy, and IST.

This center is one of the first to offer a promising new therapy called Supportive Oligonucleotide Technique (SOT), which is a gene expression therapy and does not use chemo drugs. SOT is usually only offered to patients that have no active tumors. It targets circulating cancer tumor and stem cells by inducing apoptosis, or cell death. It can also cross the blood-brain barrier.

Their website contains a number of very positive patient testimonies. The URL is: www.cancercenterforhealing.com

4. **Issels Immuno-Oncology**: Issels has an outpatient facility in Santa Barbara, California, and an inpatient Hospital in Tijuana, Mexico. It is a state-of-the-art Cancer Immunotherapy Cancer center and is designed to restore the body's own complex immune and defense mechanisms to recognize and eliminate cancer cells without the use of toxic pharmacology. They use an integrative approach with protocols that are based on years of clinical experience. They offer cancer vaccine and immune system activation protocols, advanced targeted gene therapies and hyperthermia. The Tijuana facility is used for Immunotherapy and requires patients to travel there for the vaccine to be created. Their treatment model is based on advanced therapies that are being used in Germany. Many of their metastatic patients, who failed conventional treatment, have amazing testimonies of their cancer going into remission. The URL is: www.issels.com

5. **Florida Integrative Medical Center (FIMC)**: FIMC is located in Sarasota, Florida. This center is much like the previous centers and offers an extensive menu of alternative and natural therapies that treat cancer and many other degenerative diseases. They have been in business for a number of years and have an outstanding reputation. I

can say this from first hand experience.

FIMC can also use Reflexology to help identify a more patient specific treatment plan, if a patient wishes to use it. For those who don't know what Reflexology is, let me explain.

Reflexology is an alternative medicine technique that is considered pseudoscientific by many in conventional medicine. It is based on the belief that certain pressure points on the feet hands and ears correspond to various organs and systems in the body, and that by massaging these pressure points it can benefit the health of the body. It also employs muscle response testing that uses a biofeedback loop for identifying nutritional deficiencies or sensitivities to various substances. FIMC integrates information from the Greece Tests and Reflexology to help determine the most effective substances to use. FIMC has patients from all over the southeast. The URL is: www.floridaintegrative.com

6. **Silver Institute for Life Extension Medicine**. Located in Scottsdale, AZ, Doctor Silver offers a comprehensive program of integrative and natural therapies that target cancer and other degenerative diseases. Doctor Silver is a cancer survivor himself and has been successfully treating cancer patients for over 20 years. He is also a renowned cardiologist. His personal experience brings a unique perspective to treating cancer. Like many other Alternative and Integrative Cancer Doctors he uses a whole body approach. He first preforms extensive testing in an effort to find the root causes of the disease and then develops a comprehensive treatment plan tailored to each patient's profile. He has had excellent success treating cancer patients and using IPT as a powerful integrative protocol with natural therapies. The URL is: deansilvermd.com

7. **Forsythe Cancer Care Center:** Doctor James Forsythe is a famous integrative-alternative oncologist, who has been practicing medicine for over 50 years. His clinic is in Reno, Nevada. He has successfully treated thousands of late stage cancer patients. It is astonishing that most of his patients not only go into remission, but most of them are also late stage cancer patients that have failed conventional treatment. Doctor Forsythe gives them hope and a realistic chance to survive their disease when no other option exists. Despite his success at treating late stage cancer patients, he has endured numerous vicious attacks from conventional cancer doctors and researchers.

The Forsythe Protocol is an intensive three week program of IPT sessions twice a week, and a combination of intravenous (IV) natural substance therapy on the non-IPT days. Poly-MVA is also taken orally for three or four months following the initial three-week program. Some patients might also do a once a week follow-up IPT session for up to 12 weeks while taking oral Poly-MVA. Doctor Forsythe carefully documents the outcomes of his patients. He published a 40-month study of over 500 patients with multiple types of late stage cancer, all of which participated in the IPT/Poly-MVA protocol. The average survival rate was 59 percent. In comparison to conventional treatment, his success rate is stunning.

To see the clinical results using this protocol go to URL: http://www.centurywellness.com/main-news/309-forsythe-protocol-poly-mva. For general information go to URL: drforsythe.com

8. **The Center for Advanced Medicine**: Located just north of Atlanta in Johns Creek, Georgia. Doctor Jonathan Stegall is an integrative oncologist and offers a number of popular alternative cancer therapies, including his own protocol, which is something similar to the Forsythe protocol. He also uses the Greece Tests to target each patient's cancer cells more effectively using chemo and natural substances. There are very few doctors in the southeast region of the United States who offer a comprehensive IPT and natural substance program. The URL is: drstegall.com

9. **Progressive Medical Center (PMC):** PMC is located on the north side of Atlanta, Georgia. During most of 2017, PMC offered a comprehensive cancer treatment program patterned after the Forsythe IPT protocol, however, their Integrative Oncologist left and it is uncertain as to whether they will re-staff this position in 2018. Although IPT may not be currently available, they do offer a wide range of holistic and natural therapies that target cancer and other degenerative diseases.

Like most other centers, PMC has Naturopathic Doctors and other specialists on staff. They also offer the Greece tests for targeted oral and IV therapy. The URL is: www.progressivemedicalcenter.com

10. **The Burzynski Patient Group**: Located in Houston, Texas. Doctor Stanislaw Burzynski is a prominent physician and biochemist,

who pioneered an innovative cancer therapy using targeted active peptides, called antineoplastons. His approach identifies abnormal genes and pathways that can be targeted with substances that can selectively kill cancer. Gene targeted therapy blocks the growth of cancer and does not harm healthy cells.

His patients are predominantly late stage cancer patients that failed conventional treatment, yet his patients experience a very high response rate of 40 to 60 percent. This statistic includes both partial and complete responses.[20] His greatest successes appear to be in treating brain and breast cancer, and non-Hodgkins Lymphoma. The URL is: www.burzynskipatientgroup.org

11. **Oasis of Hope Hospital**: Although Oasis of Hope Hospital is not in the United States it is worth mentioning. It is just across the border from San Diego, California in Tijuana, Mexico. It offers numerous integrative, holistic and alternative cancer therapies, some of which are not available in the United States. They publish detailed statistics on patient treatment outcomes for each type of cancer on their website and their success in treating late staged cancers is excellent. The research supporting their integrative approach is well documented on their website. The URL is: www.oasisofhope.com

12. **NORI Protocol**: NORI stands for Nutritional Oncology Research Institute. It is an independent research organization. NORI was formed by a group of researchers who put their findings together to form an alternative cancer treatment protocol. This protocol is non-toxic, low cost, safe and can be done at home. However, a certified doctor, who is trained in this protocol, is required to oversee the treatment.

The NORI Protocol targets the metabolic abnormalities found in cancer, and it emphasizes a low methionine diet. It requires patient's to take a lot of digestive enzymes. It also incorporates high dose selenium, in the form of sodium selenite, with several other natural substances that synergistically work together with a low methionine diet to cause cancer cell suicide.

To be effective, this protocol requires patients who are willing to exercise exceptional eating discipline. Of note, over exposure to selenium can be very toxic and should only be done under the supervision of a doctor. NORI also provides helpful information to their patients on how to work through the complex web of alternative

224

cancer treatment centers and how to make the best decision for their situation. To join NORI each member pays a one-time fee and must be under the care of a NORI network doctor. The URL for NORI is: https://noriprotocol.com

13. Health and Wellness Center of Carmel (HWC): HWC is located in Carmel, Indiana. WHC offers a comprehensive assortment of natural and holistic cancer therapies similar to many of the centers previously discussed.

Dr. Clifford Fetters is the Medical Director and is a national leader in holistic cancer treatment. HWC is also one of the few alternative cancer centers in the United States that offers IST. They also offer SOT for those with a low cancer load. The URL is: http://www.hwofc.com/

14. Clinic Solutions International (CSI): CSI is located in Houston, Texas and is headed by Doctor Virginia Werner, who has a Ph.D. in Nutritional Therapy. She is well versed in nutrition, biochemistry and epigenetics. Epigenetics is a field of medical science that restores damaged genes that have mutated as a result of toxins, cancer, viruses, bacteria, nutritional deficiencies, or from some other source. CSI's treatment goal is to use past and present research, and clinical experience to bring forth a healthy cellular state in the body.

They offer a unique Cellular Stress Assessment test utilizing DNA specimens from a patient's saliva. These tests help decode numerous diseases and provide a link to some cancers, endocrine disorders, allergies, yeast and fungal infections, chronic autoimmune disorders, mental illnesses, autism, dyslexia, ADD and many other degenerative conditions. They also test for the presence of over 2,000 different toxic substances, including things like parasites, metals, pesticides, and radiation damage. They use these tests to tailor a specific nutritional and herbal supplemental treatment plan that seeks to detoxify and heal the body. They might also prescribe a modified protein solution that can repair damaged genes and restore gene processes that help the body heal. In some instances Doctor Werner can restore damaged genes to the extent that it will reverse a degenerative disease, including some cancers.

Testimonies of several cancer patients are published on Doctor Werner's website. It appears Doctor Werner has had some excellent success treating Breast Cancer patient's with the BRAC1 or BAC2 gene.

Although there are not a lot of testimonies form cancer patients on this website, their protocol might help those who's immune system and gene expressions are severely damaged from chemotherapy and radiation. This approach may be very helpful in not only helping the body resist any remaining cancer but help prevent a later chemo or radiation induced cancer.

The initial cost is $3,000 for a four-part evaluation that does not require an office visit. A saliva test kit is sent to the patient in the mail with instructions on how to take the tests and ship them to the lab. The four tests include, DNA Cellular Stress Assessment, Chromosome Testing, MTHFR (Methylation) Test, and a Gene Correlation and Functionality Test. Once the tests are evaluated, Doctor Werner puts together a nutritional and herbal supplement plan, which may also include a modified protein solution. Follow up tests are performed at certain intervals to evaluate the effectiveness of the treatment regimen. Costs for the follow up tests and herbal supplements might be several hundred dollars or more a month.

Also keep in mind that since epigenetics is a process of biologically repairing damaged genes and chromosomes, it can take a number of months to get results. The URL is: www.clinic-solutions-houston

Summary

There are a lot of lessons I learned from recurrent cancer. First, never let your guard down after being treated for cancer, even if you experienced a complete therapeutic response and the cancer is in remission. Second, understand the treatment options if the cancer comes back and develop a well thought out treatment approach. Third, be aggressive with surveillance tests and adding additional layers of tests. Fourth, consider getting the Greece Tests and if there is evidence of circulating cancer tumor and stem cells, then seek a treatment center that has experience targeting circulating cancer cells.

Although I intended to have an alternative cancer treatment center lined up in case there was a recurrence, I never got around to it. I did a lot of research but could never quite get my arms around what would be best for me. This was one of the chief motivating factors for writing this book—don't do what I did! We should have also been more aggressive with the endoscopies and PET scans during the second year post chemo-radiation. If I had known about the early detection blood screening tests, I would have been doing them every three to four months. This would have caught a recurrence at a much earlier stage making the prognosis more optimistic. It would have also given me an option to try an alternative therapy before going ahead with the surgery.

Those who experience a recurrent metastatic cancer, except for a miraculous few, are at a high risk of experiencing a long and painful march toward more chemo, which will ultimately fail. I don't know about you, but I refuse to spend the last days of my life shuffling in and out of doctors offices, diagnostic centers, chemo treatment facilities and clinical trials, and then end up in a hospice, forcing my family to watch me slowly die.

Patients enter into cancer treatment centers convinced they have no other option. Few understand that there are a growing number of alternative and integrative cancer treatment centers in the United States that can provide a viable option, as either a stand-alone treatment, or a complement to a conventional treatment program.

The alternative therapies and treatment centers discussed in this book afford patients a springboard from which to explore other options more thoroughly. So don't wait around any longer. Do some research and take control of your treatment plan.

One might ask whether I would have been better off having the surgery right after the chemo and radiation—so did I. Even if I had the surgery right away, the chance of recurrence was still around 40 percent. At that time I felt it was worth the risk to play a wait and see game—a game I lost. Did I really have a healing in the first place? Yes––but it only lasted two years. Does God work in this way? Yes. Do I understand why? No. What I do understand however is that being poorly informed in regard to cancer can make the difference between life and death.

As the Psalmist writes in the Bible, "wisdom is to be more desired than rubies", which includes learning from the mistakes made by others. Please learn from my mistakes!

Notes

1. "Definition of Immunotherapy," National Cancer Institute. https://www.cancer.gov/search/results (accessed October 10, 2016).

2. "Jimmy Carter's Immunotherapy Appears to Respond to Immuno therapy," American Association of Cancer Research Foundation, https://www.aacrfoundation.org/Science/Pages/jimmy-carter.aspx (accessed October 10, 2016).

3. "Advanced Melanoma Treatments have Promise for Patients," March 16, 2015, American Academy of Dermatology." https://www.aad.org/media/news-releases/advanced-melanoma-treatments-have-promise-for-patients (accessed October 10, 2016).

4. "FDA Approves First Therapeutic Cancer Vaccine," https://www.cancer.gov/about-cancer/treatment/research/first-treatment-vaccine-approved (accessed October 3, 2016)

5. "The Stem Cell Theory of Cancer," Ludwig Center, Stanford Medicine, https://med.staford.edu/ludwigcenter/overview/theory.html (accessed October 10, 2016).

6. ONCOblot Cancer Testing with Confidence. http://ONCOblot labs.com (accessed October 4, 2016).

7. "ONCOblot the Game Changing Cancer Blood Test," Medicor Cancer Centres, http://medicorcancer.com/oncoblot (accessed October 12, 2016).

8. Cancer Imaging program: Nuclear Imaging. National Cancer Institute. http:// imaging.cancer.gov/patientsandproviders/cancerimaging/ Nuclear imaging (accessed October 13, 2016).

9. Ibid, Medicor.

10. Ibid.

11. Ibid, ONCOblotlabs.com.

12. Overcoming Trastuzumab Resistance in HER2+ Esophagogastric Cancer, Memorial Sloan Kettering Cancer Center, https:// www. mskcc.org/clinical-updates/overcoming-trastuzumab-resistance-her 2-esophagogastric (accessed October 4, 2016).

13. High Dose Vitamin C (PDQ) – Patient Version. National Cancer Institute, https:// www.cancer.gov/about-cancer/treatment/cam/ patient/vitamin-c-pdq (accessed October 13, 2016).

14. Tests/Oncocount R.G.C.C., https://rgcc-group.com/index. php?page=testoncocount rgcc

15. Cologuard.http://www.cologuardtest.com/what-is-cologuard/how -effective-is-cologuard (accessed October 4, 2016).

16. Chustecka, Zosia, November 26, 2014 "High Price Tag for Cologuard Confirmed, but Test is Welcomed,"

http://www.medscape.com/viewarticle/835506
(accessed October 4, 2016).

17. American Cancer Society Guidelines for the Early Detection of Cancer. http://www.cancer.org/healthy/findcancerearly/ cancerscreeningguidelines/american-cancer-society-guidelines-for -the-early-detection-of-cancer (accessed October 4, 2016).

18. Prostate Cancer Prevention and Early Detection, http://www.cancer.org/cancer/prostatecancermoreinformation/ prostatecancerearlydetection/prostate-cancer-early-detect (accessed October 4, 2016).

19. Kavita Nanda, MD, et. al, "Accuracy of the Papanicolaou Test in Screening for and Follow-up of Cervical Cytologic Abnormalities: A Systematic Review," Annals of Internal Medicine, 16 May 2000, Vol 132, 10. http://annals.org/article.aspx?articleid=713473 (accessed October 4, 2016).

20. "Burzynski's Antineoplaston Therapy," Cancer Compass, http://cancercompass alternateroute.com/doctors-and-clinics/Stanislaw -burzynski-and-his-antineoplaston-treatment (accessed October 14, 2016).

CHAPTER 16

A Final Word

Happy is the one who finds wisdom,
the one who gains understanding!
—Proverbs 3:13, 15

To end, this book illustrates that cancer patients hold a tremendous amount of power in their hands to affect the outcome of their illness. This power can only be wielded when patients decide to take control of their treatment plan. When doing so, they become an active participant with their medical team in the healing process. Taking control of, and participating in the treatment plan makes the patient the primary stakeholder in the healing process, not the doctor; and for what better reason than to live. The holistic prescriptions investigated in this book empower the patient to live. They are scientifically founded and most of them can be safely done at home. Any cancer patient can use these antidotes to attack their cancer prior to treatment, make the treatment more effective, reduce the side effects of chemo, radiation and surgery, and help prevent recurrence. More so, when these things are combined with any type of treatment, be it conventional, integrative, alternative, or dietary, the outcomes are significantly improved as well as the quality of life. All the scientific research says so.

It's About Improving Outcomes

At a minimum, cancer patients can improve their outcome by simply fortifying their body with exercise, targeted natural substances, and an alkaline diet. If they want to attack their cancer more aggressively, and if they can summon the eating discipline to do so, they can exploit the metabolic abnormalities of cancer with diet. With that said, eating one's cancer to death is not such an easy thing to do on one's own accord. A better approach for many might be to pay out of pocket and be under the supervision of a physician associated with the NORI Protocol, or another alternative cancer treatment program. NORI or an alternative cancer doctor would also be able to attack the cancer with targeted natural supplement therapy at the same time the cancer is being stressed by diet, making it an optimal approach.

Beyond exercise, diet and natural substance therapy, an alternative cancer center can offer patients a whole host of integrative and alternative therapies, and they can bring their experience to bear with a bouquet of therapeutic approaches that are tailored to each patient's needs. In this situation, the patient is afforded multiple directions from which to attack their cancer. The biggest drawbacks to alternative therapies is not the notion that they are unsafe, rather, it is they can be somewhat expensive.

The second biggest drawback is that most patients do not possess extensive knowledge of alternative cancer therapies and treatment centers, and consequently believe they have no other option than to receive more chemo, experimental drugs or enter into a clinical trial. Hopefully, this is no longer true for those who have read this book. Patients always have options that add to, or go beyond conventional medicine that may extend their life beyond anything they imagined. The problem is very few people know about them.

Even if a patient decides to stay the course with conventional treatment, it is critical they understand that if they have a metastatic cancer, they will most likely perish. An alternative treatment center affords hope when all else seems lost.

Whatever path the patient chooses, it is prudent to consider using the Greece or ONCOblot blood tests for an additional layer of early detection—the earlier it is detected, the easier it is to treat. The Greece tests can also help doctors use targeted therapies against the cancer.

Keep in mind, it much more advantageous to have a group of specialists on your treatment team, not just your Oncologist and Internist. Five heads are much better than two when it comes to improving outcomes.

Knowledge Is Power

The idea that we can treat illness with food remains an alien concept in the minds of most Americans. Food as medicine is an ancient concept, promoted by Hippocrates, but it flies in the face of a medical system dominated by large corporations that are profit driven. Not that being profit driven is necessarily evil, it's more of a matter of a synthetically minded health delivery system serving a synthetically compliant and sheepishly dependent culture. If it is not copyrightable it's not going to be put on the playing field. The only group of losers in this scenario is the patients. In the American mindset, medicine is drugs, and food is food—period. Unless this roadblock is removed in a cancer patient's mind, it is questionable as to whether they will ever swallow the food as medicine concept presented in this book. The elixir for this ailment is scientifically backed studies that prove food and natural substances can prevent, attack and even kill cancer. Unless this knowledge is made known to a much wider audience, many more will continue to perish prematurely, much to the disgrace of the 40 plus year war on cancer.

The same roadblock with food also exists with the concept of alternative cancer treatment centers. Like me initially, most people do not have a clue about them. We all fear the unknown as much as anything else. The only palatable remedy is to feed an interested patient a plate full of scientifically flavored knowledge. All of these things speak directly to me. My whole cancer story is peppered with doing a number of wrong things with diet and lifestyle far too long, and doing a number of right things far too late. I went on a sabbatical because I knew my stressful job was pushing me over the edge, only to discover that this sound remedy was a tad late. My response to the crisis seemed to always be a half step behind. I would have never gotten into this predicament in the first place, if I had known about the strong link between chronic acid reflux and cancer. It makes me surmise that Thomas Gray's pithy statement in his poem *Ode To A Distant Prospect Of Eaton College*, "ignorance is bliss," is not so pithy—because my ignorance almost killed me. I also wish I had known a lot more about how to prevent recurrence, early detection cancer blood tests and where to get them, how to attack the metabolic weaknesses of cancer with diet, and alternative cancer therapies and treatment centers. There you have it, the cornerstones of this book.

The point is—the better informed we become, the wiser we can be in pursuing a treatment plan that affords us the best possible opportunity to live longer and have a better quality of life.

In Retrospect

If I had known the things that I know now, I never would have gone through with high dose chemo-radiation, or the surgery. I would have started with the Hybrid Cancer Diet and intravenous natural substance therapy, followed by other alternative or integrative therapies, if needed, including IPT. If that failed, I would consider surgery as an absolute last option. Be that as it may, I am not telling anyone to opt out of conventional therapy. I am simply expressing what I believe would have been the best approach for me, because conventional therapy took a devastating toll on my body and my life in general. In spite of all the treatments, all of the suffering, all of the damage done to my body and quality of life, I remain in a high risk category for recurrence. Yes, I am thankful that I am alive—but at what cost? The system is miserably broken.

A Final Word

I am reminded of the day we packed up our cars and drove to Bradenton Beach in September 2013, expecting a sabbatical time of rest from the burdens of life, but instead, I found myself in a fight for my life that has gone on for the better part of five years. I am however, grateful that I fell ill that day, otherwise the tumor would have been discovered too late. Kelly has been in the midst of this fight as well and has shouldered a very difficult burden. Passing through the furnace of affliction is difficult, but it has made us both better people. The fire is indeed hot, but the perseverance in faith that it produces is priceless. I lost a number of things during this journey, as most cancer patients' do, and so did my wife. Yet, in a strange way, I gained other things that are intrinsically more valuable. The cancer may have taken away my good health—but it was replaced with better nutrition and eating habits. It may have taken away my well-crafted plans for the future—but it showed me how to rest and be at peace with my life, no matter what the circumstance. Most remarkably, it awakened in my heart a greater realization that my misfortune cannot deny me the true happiness of the Kingdom of God, or a sabbatical rest beyond anything this world can offer

EPILOGUE

Shortly after releasing the first edition of Volume I, I was diagnosed with a single metastatic liver tumor. This came as no surprise, since the Oncocount tests showed elevated circulating cancer tumor and stem cells throughout the prior year. During this period I was not physically strong enough to enter into an alternative treatment program due to the horrific complications of the esophagectomy. The words of my oncologist at MD Anderson echoed in my ear again, "If you have a recurrence after the surgery there is no cure for you [you will die]." Metastatic esophageal cancer––so it goes, comes with a dismal survival rate. Maybe 2 percent if you're lucky—but the story does not end here.

The good news, if there could be such a thing, was that a single metastatic lesion in the liver is uncommon. My oncologist said, "There is an improved chance of survival if treated with maximum dose chemo following the surgery." He insisted that maximum dose chemo would provide my best chance of survival—and so did my Internist. I said, "Thanks, but no thanks." I asked my oncologist if he could do fractionalized chemo, and he said, "No, it is not part of the standard of care." "Here we go again," I thought. Low dose, and less harmful use of FDA approved chemo drugs remains on the black list of the mind-numb chemo robots of conventional therapy.

Then I was offered Keytruda, the darling Immunotherapy drug of oncologists. Keytruda is touted as a breakthrough drug, but has only been effective in putting several types of cancers into remission. It's side effects can be serious and even life threatening. It's one of those drugs they've been advertising on TV for years now, with the typical mind-conditioning ploy used in most drug commercials. It starts off with a handsome middle-aged couple strolling down a breathtaking park trail, something akin to the opening scene of the *Sound Of Music*. They wistfully glance into each other's eyes as a voice similar to James Earl Jones invites us to embrace a certain drug, with all of its side effects. All the while enchanting piano music plays in the background. Who can resist. Our hearts melt. The dreadful list of side effects they just read to us do not really seem that bad anymore. It's sort of like smiling at someone while you haul off and smack'em. The problem with Keytruda and me, other than the side effects, is not that I don't like the opening scene of the Sound of Music, it's that my cancer cells were tested and showed zero sensitivity to it. Alas, what are we do to with somebody like Maria?

After my dance with Keytruda they offered me a shot at a Phase II clinical trial. Fat chance! I made up my mind on clinical trials long ago—in a galaxy far, far away. Come on? This was the third time I was diagnosed with cancer—don't you think I'd get a little smarter each time? I would rather go on a water fast for a week and run five miles a day than be a lab rat in a clinical trail.

Instead of conventional treatment, I entered into a four-week alternative-integrative treatment program at Progressive Medical Center in Atlanta, which uses IPT and is patterned after the James Forsythe protocol. After this program the circulating cancer cells dropped from 6.5 to 5.2. Normal is considered less than 5, but in many instances cancer will still grow in a new location unless this number drops down to less than 2. The PET and CT scans showed no evidence of metastatic disease.

Over the next 10 months I did a number of oral and IV natural substance therapies, along with three more IPT infusions, a semi-low methionine diet, and regular exercise, hoping it would bring the cell count below 5—but it didn't work. The cell count remained slightly elevated. I recently entered IST and remain optimistic that this will have a positive impact. I also added epigenetics as a complement to the immunotherapy.

All of my doctors are surprised and delighted at my progress—so is my family—and so am I.

APPENDIX A

Foods By LEVEL of pH

Alkaline	More Neutral	Acidic
Asparagus	Almond Milk	Animal Proteins
Beans – all types	Almonds	Beef
Beets	Apples	Bison
Broccoli	Apricots	Chicken
Brussel Sprouts	Bananas	Clams
Cabbage	Blueberry	Crabs
Carrots	Cantaloupe	Eggs
Cauliflower	Cherries	Fish - ocean
Cayenne Pepper	Coconut	Liver, and other
Celery	Corn	organs
Cucumber	Cranberry	Lobster
Dandelion	Currants	Pork Veal
Endive	Dates	Sugars
Garlic	Fish - Freshwater	Artificial
Green Beans	Gooseberry	Sweeteners
Horseradish	Grapes	Barley Malt Syrup
Kohlrabi	Kidney Beans	Beet Sugar
Leeks	Mango	Brown Rice Syrup
Lettuce	Oranges	Cane Sugar
Lentils	Papaya	Chocolate
Onions	Peaches	High Fructose
Peas	Pears	Corn Syrup
Red Cabbage	Pineapple	Ice Cream
Rhubarb	Plums	Rice Sugar
Rutabaga	Potatoes	Beverages
Soy Nuts	Raspberry	Alcohol
Spinach	Rose Hips	Beer, Wine
Tofu	Sweet Potatoes	Coffee

Alkaline	More Neutral	Acidic
Turnip	Strawberry	Sodas
Watercress	Tangerine	Sweetened Juices
Zucchini	Watermelon	Tea – Black
Fruits	Sugars	Nuts
Avocado	Raw Honey	Cashews
Fresh Lemon	Maple Syrup	Peanuts
Grapefruit	Molasses	Pecans
Limes	Nuts	Pistachios
Olives	Brazil Nuts	Dairy
Tomatoes	Sesame & Sunflower	Hard Cheese
Nuts	Seeds	Cream
Almonds	Walnuts	Bread/Grains
Hazelnuts	Dairy	White
	Cottage Cheese	Biscuits
	Cream Cheese	Pasta
	Goat Cheese	White Rice Flour
	Milk	Condiments
	Sour Cream	Ketchup
	Yogurt	Mayo
	Bread/Grains	Mustard
	Whole grains	Salad Dressings
	Oils	Soy Sauce
	Butter	Miscellaneous
	Coconut	Canned Fruit
	Corn	Navy Beans
	Flaxseed	Pinto Beans
	Margarine	White Rice
	Olive	
	Sunflower	

APPENDIX B

Staging Cancer

A. Background

Staging and treatment of any cancer is a complex process that requires a number of diagnostic tests and/or biopsies, and careful evaluation to determine how far a disease is advanced. Accurate Staging allows the doctor to apply an appropriate Standard of Care (SOC) for treatment. It is extremely helpful to understand staging and the treatment options of cancer, so please take time to study your disease. This appendix describes staging for cancer in general, and also provides a list of helpful websites that explain staging and treatment more specifically for esophageal cancer.

B. Staging

Stage refers to how far advanced the cancer is, such as the size of the tumor, and how far it has spread to local or distant areas. Knowing the stage of the cancer helps the doctor determine the following better:
– How serious the cancer is and the chance of survival.
– The best course of treatment.
– Other potential treatment options, such as a clinical trial.

A cancer is always referred to by the stage it was given at diagnosis, even if it gets worse or spreads. New information about how a cancer has changed over time gets added on to the original stage. So, the stage doesn't change, even though the cancer might.

How Stage Is Determined: To learn the stage of the disease, the doctor may order x-rays, lab tests, and other tests or procedures.

Systems that Describe Staging: There are many staging systems. For example, the TNM staging system is used for many types of cancer. Others are specific to a particular type of cancer.

Most staging systems include information about:
– Where the tumor is located in the body.
– The cell type, such as, adenocarcinoma or squamous cell.
– The size of the tumor.
– Whether the cancer has spread to nearby lymph nodes.
– Whether the cancer has spread to a different part of the body.
– Tumor grade, which refers to how abnormal the cancer cells look, its metabolic rate, and how likely the tumor is to grow and spread.

C. The TNM Staging System
(Source: http://www.cancer.gov/about-cancer/diagnosis-staging/ staging)

The TNM system is the most widely used cancer staging system. Most hospitals and medical centers use the TNM system as their main method for cancer reporting. Most cancer patients are likely to see their cancer described by this staging system in their pathology report, unless they have a cancer for which a different staging system is used. Examples of cancers with different staging systems include brain and spinal cord tumors, and blood cancers.

TNM system:
The **T** refers to the size and extent of the main tumor. The main tumor is called the primary tumor.
The **N** refers to the number of nearby lymph nodes that have cancer.
The **M** refers to whether the cancer has metastasized. This means that the cancer has spread from the primary tumor to other parts of the body.

When the cancer is described by the TNM system, there will be numbers after each letter that give more detail about the cancer. For example, T1N0MX or T3N1M0. The following explains what the letters and numbers mean:

Primary tumor (T)

TX: Main tumor cannot be measured.

T0: Main tumor cannot be found.

T1, T2, T3, T4: Refers to the size and/or extent of the main tumor. The higher the number after the T, the larger the tumor or the more it has grown into nearby tissues. T's may be further divided to provide more detail, such as T3a and T3b.

Regional lymph nodes (N)

NX: Cancer in nearby lymph nodes cannot be measured.

N0: There is no cancer in nearby lymph nodes.

N1, N2, N3: Refers to the number and location of lymph nodes that contain cancer. The higher the number after the N, the more lymph nodes involved.

Distant metastasis (M)

MX: Metastasis cannot be measured.

M0: Cancer has not spread to other parts of the body.

M1: Cancer has spread to other parts of the body.

D. Links

1. Staging (TNM) – Esophageal Cancer
http://www.cancer.org/cancer/esophaguscancer/detailedguide/
esophagus-cancer-staging
http://www.doctorslounge.com/oncology/tnm/esophagus.htm

2. Treatment and General Information – Esophageal Cancer
http://www.cancer.gov/cancertopics/pdq/treatment/esophageal/
HealthProfessional/page3
http://www.cancer.gov/cancertopics/pdq/treatment/esophageal/
health-professional
http://www.medicinenet.com/esophageal_cancer/article.htm

Appendix C

Methionine Content In Food
(To be used with the Hybrid Cancer Diet)

Source
U.S. Department of Agriculture, Food Consumption Data Base
Search more foods at URL: www.https://ndb.nal.usda.gov/ndb/search/list

Amount of Methionine in mg, per 100 grams, or 3.5 ounces of food			
Food	Methionine	Food	Methionine
Egg White, Dried Power (glucose reduced) 3204		Chicken, grilled 794	
Cod fish, dried and salted 1859		Swiss Cheese 792	
Sesame Flour, low-fat 1656		Swiss Cheese 784	
Egg, whole, dried 1477		Parmesan Cheese, grated 751	
Seaweed, Spirulina, dried 1149		Pumpkin, Squash seeds 740	
Soy Protein, isolate 1130		Corned Beef 711	
Cheese, Parmesan, shredded 1114		Tuna, white, canned 700	
Sunflower Seed flour 1043		Soy Flour 634	
Cheese, Parmesan, grated 1016		Tofu, dry, frozen 613	
Brazil Nuts, dried 1008		Salmon 631	
Parmesan Cheese, dry 971		American Cheese, processed 579	
Skim Milk, powder 907		Cheddar Cheese 547	
Beef Chuck, cooked, braised 897		Alaskan King Crab 545	
Beef Round, cooked, braised 894		Black Walnuts 479	
Turkey, wing meat, cooked 893		Ground Beef, 85% lean 572	
Milk, dry, non-fat 890		Egg White 394	
Beef Brisket, lean, cooked 883		Whole Boiled Egg 392	
Tuna, canned light 862		Pistachio Nuts 386	
Watermelon Seeds, dried 833		Brown Rice, medium gr. cooked 321	
Cheese, Gruyere 822		Peanuts 289	
Pork, ham, cooked 819		Walnuts, English 286	
Chicken, light meat, cooked 815		White flour, enriched 283	
Soy Protein, concentrate 814		Peanut Butter 262	
Goat Cheese, hard 813		Cereals, wheat, ready to eat 257	
Turkey, all classes, cooked 811		Cheerios Cereal 254	
Beef, sirloin 795		Oatmeal 250	
		Fava Beans 239	

Amount of Methionine in mg, per 100 grams, or 3.5 ounces of food	
Food Methionine	Food Methionine
Mixed Nuts 228	Baked Beans, canned 57
Rice Flour 228	Cereals, Quick Oats, cooked 46
Soybeans 224	Rice Noodles, cooked 43
Barley 208	Mushrooms, raw 40
Tofu, firm 202	Avocado, raw 39
Grape Nuts Cereal 200	Broccoli, raw 38
Pecans, dry roasted 189	Coconut Milk 38
Quinoa, cooked 178	Sweet Potato, cooked 37
Wheaties Cereal 168	Kale, raw 36
Tortilla chips, white corn 167	Cream of Wheat, corn, cooked 34
Almonds, dry roasted & Yogurt 155	Figs, dried 34
English Muffins, whole wheat 154	Sweet Potato, canned 32
Bread, cracked wheat 148	Cream of Chicken Soup 33
White Beans 146	Potato, baked 31
Black Turtle Beans 141	Asparagus 31
Navy Beans 131	Amaranth 31
Kidney Beans, red 130	Grits, corn 30
Almond Butter 122	Mushrooms, cooked 30
Wild Rice, cooked 119	Cauliflower, cooked 28
Chickpeas, Garbanzo 116	Soy Milk 27
Black-eyed Peas 110	Kelp 25
White Rice, long gr. 100	Chicken Vegetable Soup
Lima Beans 100	(canned) 25
Pasta, whole wheat, cooked 97	Mustard Greens 25
Mixed Vegetables 93	Tomatoes 24
Pinto Beans, canned, cooked 85	Red Potatoes 24
Millet 85	Cream of Potato Soup, canned 24
Whole Milk 83	Peppers, hot, red, chili, green 24
Pop Corn (cheese popcorn 181) 83	Kiwi 24
Green Peas, frozen, cooked 78	Brussel Sprouts 24
Lentils 77	Apricots 24
Corn, cooked 70	Mayonnaise, with egg 23
White Rice, long-gr. (cooked) 63	Macadamia Nuts, dry roasted 23
Oats, in cereal 60	Yam 23
Pasta, gluten free 59	Beans, Green, Yellow, Snap 23
Brown Rice, long gr., cooked 58	Dates 22
Spinach, cooked 55	Instant Coffee, Decaf 22
Brown Rice, cooked 53	Cabbage 22

Amount of Methionine in mg, per 100 grams, or 3.5 ounces of food			
Food	**Methionine**	**Food**	**Methionine**
Coleslaw	22	Pickles	10
Rice Noodles, cooked	21	Cherries	10
Seedless Raisins	21	Bananas	8
Sweet Potatoes, cooked	21	Plums	8
Grapes, raw	21	Tomato Sauce, canned	8
Butter	21	Chicken Broth, Swanson	8
Okra	20	Squash, cooked	7
Cauliflower, raw	20	Arrow Root flour	6
Carrots, raw	20	Cucumber, raw, peeled	6
Swiss Chard	20	Watermelon	6
Turnips	20	Grapefruit	6
Tomato Paste	19	Salad Dressing, Italian	6
Kale, cooked	18	Nectarines	6
Beets	18	Melons	6
Tomato Soup	18	Mangos	5
Minestrone Soup	18	Celery	5
Tomato Products, canned	18	Apricots, dried	5
Zucchini	17	Tomato Juice	4
Iceberg Lettuce, leafy greens	16	Orange Juice	3
Romaine	16	Apple	2
Guavas	16	Papayas	2
Oranges	15	Pears	2
Peaches	15	Strawberries	1
Olives, canned, bottled	14	Coffee, brewed, tap water	0
Carrots	14	Tea, black, brewed, tap water	0
Salad Dressings, Russian	13	Table Wine	0
Pumpkin, canned	13	Beer, regular	0
Blueberries	12	Syrups	0
Cucumber, unpeeled	12	Tea, green	0
Pineapple	11	Wheat Germ	0
Eggplant	10	Vinegar	0
Onion	10	Mayonnaise, without egg	0
Peaches	10	Vegetable Oils (all)	0

General Notes:

1. All concentrated animal based proteins, especially dried proteins, such as meats, fish and cheese, have very high concentrations of methionine, and should be avoided.

2. When foods are cooked or canned, there is typically a loss of methionine.

3. Fruits contain very low levels of methionine, and not far behind are vegetables.

4. Plant based oils contain zero methionine. However, fat consumption should be kept low to moderate, because too much fat can cause insulin resistance, which might accelerate the growth of the cancer.

5. From the above list, one can monitor their daily intake of methionine, and develop a fairly well balanced Hybrid Cancer Diet with a combination of fruits, vegetables, juices, and plant based oils.

The diet can be supplemented periodically with nuts, such as macadamia and almonds, as well as, legumes, lentils and small portions of oatmeal.

6. Refer to Chapter 7 for the clinical study that demonstrated that it was safe to sustain a low methionine diet for an extended period. It this study, patients were safely restricted to 0.9 mg/1 pound of weight, per daily. For example, for some one weighing 150 pounds, restrict consumption to 140 mg.

Shorter and more intense restriction of methionine is possible for those who are not compromised with other serious health issues.

Going on a water only fast for one to two days, prior to starting this diet, would be extremely beneficial in detoxifying the body and bring methionine levels down quickly.

7. Always consult with a physician before making any significant changes to diet, especially when in a cancer treatment program.

8. When using the above table, remember, the values for methionine are for a 3.5-ounce portion of that particular food, which is pretty close to a half of a cup.

9. Enjoy eating your cancer to death!

248

Appendix D

FRUITS BY LEVEL OF SUGAR
Very Low in Sugar Avocados Limes Lemons Olives Rhubarb
Low in Sugar Cranberries Grapefruit Guavas Papaya Strawberries Tomatoes Watermelon
Medium in Sugar Apricots Blackberries Blueberries Cantaloupe Cherries (sour) Figs Melons - Honey Nectarines Peaches Plums Raspberries Tangerines

High in Sugar
Apples
Kiwifruit
Oranges
Pears
Pineapple
Pomegranates

Very High in Sugar
Apples
Bananas
Cherries (sweet)
Mangos

Highest in Sugar
Dried Fruits (because of dehydration)
Apricots
Dates
Figs
Prunes
Raisins
Canned Fruits (corn syrup added)
Sour Fruits (sugar infused)

INDEX

A

B

C

F

G

H

I

Myelodysplastic Syndrome, 190

N

National Cancer Institute, 45, 60, 73,
92, 98, 119, 129, 134, 143, 155,
158, 202, 228
National Institute of Health, 24, 39, 47,
57, 85, 143, 150
Naturopathic doctor, 147
Naturopathic Doctors, 58, 105, 147,
223
naturopathic medicine, 92, 193
NDV, 206, 207
NDV-DC vaccine, 206
neuropathy, 154, 174, 187, 190
neurotoxicity, 207
Newcastle Disease Virus, 206
Nexium, 21
Nightshade Plants, 47, 55
NIH, 47, 53, 151
Nitrates, 71
nitrites, 71, 72
nitrosamines, 71, 72, 73, 74, 77, 78
non-Hodgkins Lymphoma, 57
Non-Small Cell Lung Cancer, 151, 158
Nori Protocol, 111, 224, 232
NSCLC, 151, 153, 158, 203
nutritional excess, 62, 63
Nutritional Therapy, 225
Nutritionist, 116
Nutritionists, 129

O

Oasis of Hope Hospital, 224
obesity, 20, 45, 61, 64, 99, 134, 135,
143
Omega 3's, 52, 106
Omega 6's, 52
Omega 9, 52, 106
ONCOblot test, 209, 210
Otto H. Warburg, 100, 101
Ovarian cancer, 20
oxygen therapy, 102, 105

P

Pancreatic cancer, 169

pancreatic enzymes, 130, 147, 148, 149
Pancreatin, 148
PAP test, 215
PEMF, 190, 220
peptides, 207, 223
Periodic Fasting, 185
pesticides, 49, 50, 69, 72, 75, 100
PET scan, 83, 89, 103, 130, 177, 197,
209
pH, 77
pH strips, 171
pharynx, 9, 22, 29, 40
pH-chemistry, 66
photodynamic therapy, 33
Phyto-Sitosterols, 192
Pneuma-Zyme, 191
Poly-MVA, 214, 222
polyphenols, 152
poor nutrition, 61
positive attitude, 84, 85, 93, 125, 126,
133
Post Treatment Exercise, 140
potential hydrogen, 65
PPI, 11, 28, 32, 37, 38
PPI's, 32, 37
precursor drugs, 125
President Jimmy Carter, 203
preventing cancer, 68, 151, 204
Prilosec, 21
Probiotics, 63, 186
Progressive Medical Center, 223, 237
Propofol, 7, 179
prostate cancer, 109, 136, 154, 168,
215
prostate carcinoma, 154
prostrate cancer, 109, 148, 155
Proton Pump Inhibitor, 11
proton pump inhibitors, 37
Proton Therapy, 129
Protonix, 11
PSA, 109, 210, 215
PSA test, 215
Psoriasis, 57
Pulsed Electro-Magnetic Force, 190

Q

quercetin, 151, 152

V

vegetable, 196
vigorous-intensity exercise, 134
Vitamin C, 67, 147, 152, 155, 194,
  213, 220, 228
Vitamin D3, 147, 148, 214
voice box and throat cancer, 17

W

water-only fast, 115
Wayne State University, 167
Weill Medical College, 151
white blood cells, 45, 67, 99, 136, 151,
  193, 205, 206

Z

Zantac, 21

ABOUT THE AUTHOR

Joseph Marx has a B.A from George Washington University, and a M.S. from the University of Colorado, Boulder's Center for Advanced Training in Engineering and Computer Science and an extensive background in technical research, writing and speaking. As a former Navy Officer he served as a Navy Flight Officer, and also worked as an Intelligence Research-Analyst, Briefer, and Aerospace Engineer. He worked at Bellcore and Lucent Technologies as a Senior Consultant and Systems Engineer, and authored various White Papers, Business Requirements and Design documents for multi-services networks, and spoke at Industry wide conferences. He is also a former High School Science and Mathematics Teacher and Adjunct College Instructor. He prides himself in the ability to take complex topics and break them down in easy to understand ways. He has four children and lives with his wife Kelly in Florida. His hobbies include reading, exercising, sailing, fishing, hiking and international travel.

Joseph Marx
Victoryovercancer.org

www.ingramcontent.com/pod-product-compliance
Lightning Source LLC
Chambersburg PA
CBHW072119270326
41931CB00010B/1606